Yoga *for* Wimps

YOGA

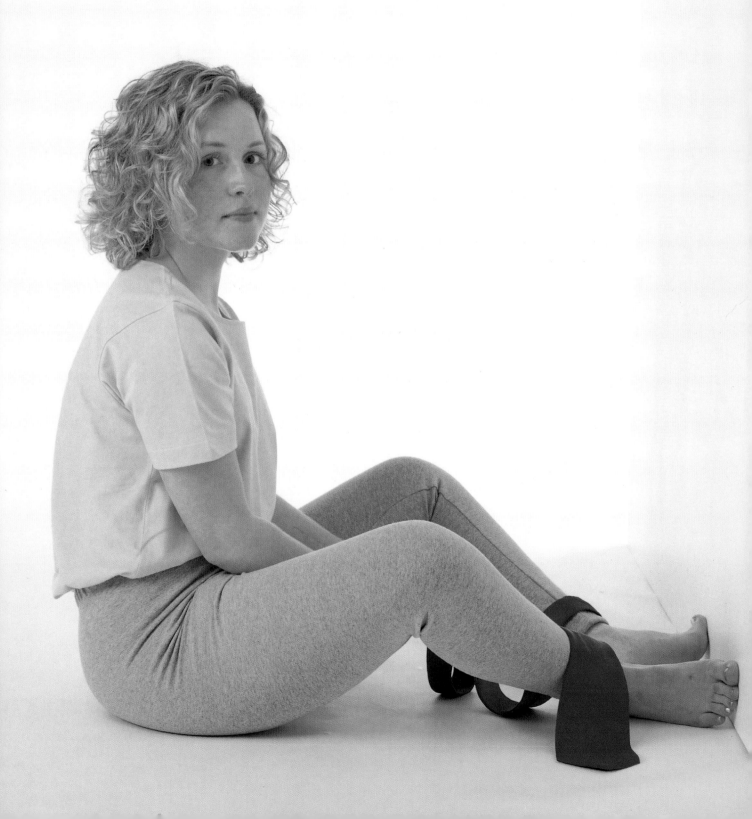

for WIMPS

POSES FOR

THE FLEXIBLY

IMPAIRED

Miriam Austin

Photography by Barry Kaplan

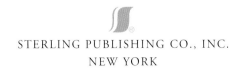

STERLING PUBLISHING CO., INC.

NEW YORK

Art direction and design by Lubosh Cech
Photography by Barry Kaplan

This book is not intended to replace expert medical advice. The author and the publisher urge you to verify the appropriateness of any procedure or exercise with your qualified health care professional. The author and the publisher disclaim any liability or loss, personal or otherwise, resulting from the procedures and information in this book.

Library of Congress Cataloging-in-Publication Data
20 19 18 17 16 15 14 13 12

Published by Sterling Publishing Co., Inc.
387 Park Avenue South, New York, N.Y. 10016
© 2000 by Miriam Austin
Distributed in Canada by Sterling Publishing
c/o Canadian Manda Group, One Atlantic Avenue, Suite 105
Toronto, Ontario, Canada M6K 3E7
Distributed in Great Britain by Chrysalis Books
64 Brewery Road, London N7 9NT, England
Distributed in Australia by Capricorn Link (Australia) Pty Ltd.
P.O. Box 704, Windsor, NSW 2756 Australia

Printed in Hong Kong

Sterling ISBN 0-8069-4339-4

You can visit Miriam Austin at her website:
www.yogaforwimps.com

To my dear sister Angie, who could never touch her toes
but who touched everyone's heart.

Acknowledgments

Having now written a book, I know why every author thanks so many people. A book is truly a group project. Thanks to everyone at Sterling who worked on this book, many of whom I have not met and many whose names I don't even know. A particular thanks to those I do know — Lincoln Boehm, Charles Nurnberg, Rachel Gaffney, Lubosh Cech, and Barry Kaplan.

Great thanks to my literary agent, Paula Balzer, of the Stuart Krichevsky Literary Agency, for her enthusiasm, for her guidance, and most important, for her friendship.

Thanks to my dear friend Melissa Hardy for assistance on the proposal.

I particularly want to thank Nancy Crum Stechert, my first yoga teacher. Nancy at times allowed me to "wimp out" and at other times encouraged me out of my wimpiness. I cannot thank Nancy enough for her love and commitment to me, both as a friend and as a teacher.

Nancy's teachers, B.K.S. Iyengar and Ramanand Patel, are responsible for most of the poses in this book. Mr. Iyengar's contributions to yoga have changed the lives of millions of people throughout the world. Yoga would not be what it is today without Mr. Iyengar's ingenuity. For several years, I was regularly blessed with Ramanand's genius. His expertise, his sense of humor, and his commitment to his students are beyond measure.

And thanks to all of my other teachers, particularly Francie Ricks and Bonnie Anthony, whom I studied with regularly in Pasadena.

With deep love and gratitude, I thank my husband Van for his encouragement, and sometimes insistence, that I transform my dream into reality.

Most important, I want to thank the Divine Power that brought yoga into my life.

Contents

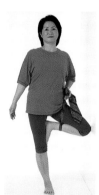

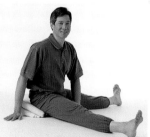

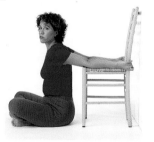

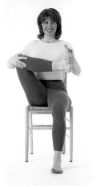

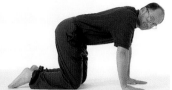

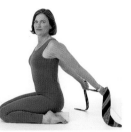

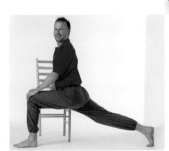

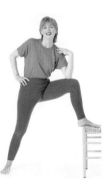

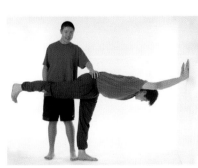

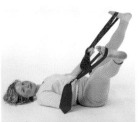

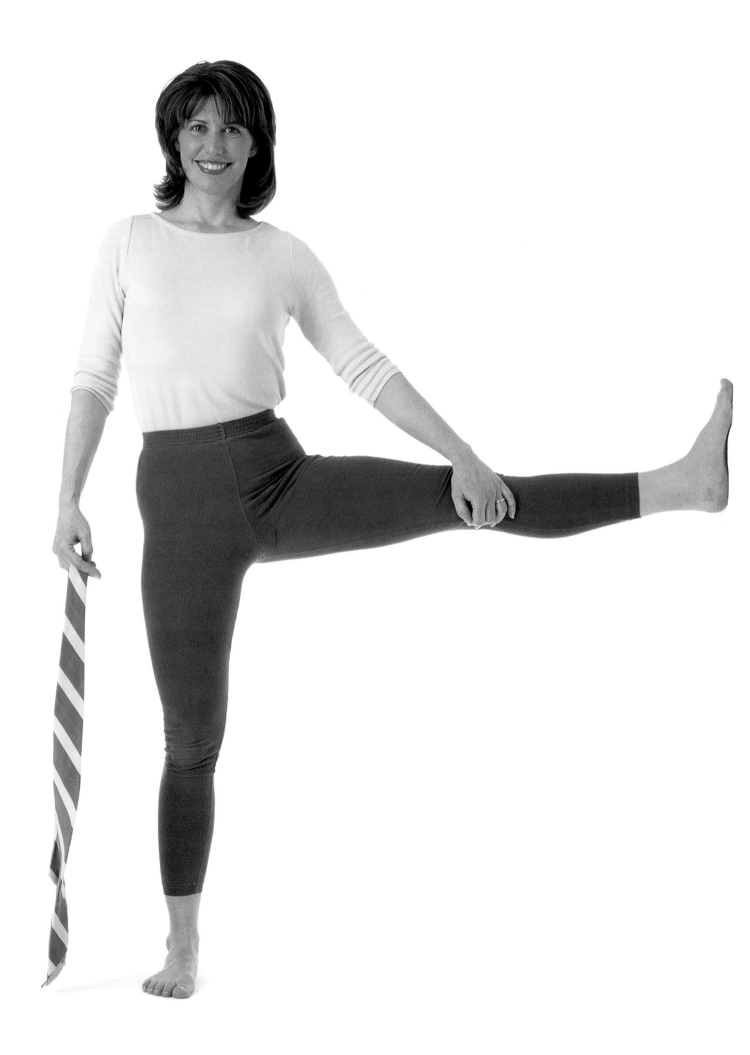

Author's Preface

Yoga is currently very popular — and rightly so! It is a terrific discipline designed to heal the body and vitalize the spirit. In recent years, movie stars as well as professional yoga teachers have bombarded us with their versions of the best postures. They make the most difficult poses look effortless, enticing us to try this ancient art that promises to transform our bodies as well as our souls. But there is one thing they are not telling us: yoga is very, very difficult and most of us cannot possibly do the demonstrated poses.

Yoga for Wimps is different. It is for the vast majority of us who are not very strong or flexible, and yet would like to be able to do yoga to help reduce stress, relieve lower back pain, enhance our athletic pursuits, or reclaim our general sense of well-being. The postures profiled in *Yoga for Wimps* are physically challenging, yet can be done by the average person. In fact, many of the postures are preliminary yoga poses. Regular practice of these poses will prepare our bodies for doing the traditional, more difficult poses, or we can simply practice the poses in *Yoga for Wimps* and reap the rewards yoga promises *right now*.

I started practicing yoga in 1986. At the time, I was an investment advisor and an avid runner, bicyclist, and skier. Through a friend, I met a yoga teacher, Nancy Crum, who had me doing backbends on her kitchen floor

the very first night we met. I felt terrific! Nancy was not teaching at that time, so I took classes from other teachers and found the beginner classes so difficult that I quickly sustained several injuries. Shortly thereafter, I quit taking classes and practiced the few poses I knew at home.

About a year later, I had a knee and lower back injury, resulting in surgery. I could no longer run or bicycle. So I went back to yoga, in search of a teacher who could help me with my physical problems, give me a good workout, and not injure me in the process. Fortunately, Nancy had just opened a yoga school. I fully committed to yoga and found that my back pain disappeared the days I did yoga and reappeared the days I didn't. Even more astounding was that within eight months something "clicked" in my hip and I have had no knee pain since. That was in 1988.

As time went on, I began to experience some of the other benefits of yoga. Not long after starting to practice yoga, I took a job in Los Angeles. I got up each morning at 4:30 a.m. to practice yoga before the 6:30 opening of the New York Stock Exchange. My incentive was not just a pain-free back — I was more calm, more centered, and able to make better investment decisions. Many colleagues said they always knew which days I practiced yoga and which days I didn't — it reflected in my trading.

In addition to all of these benefits, I was impressed with yoga's practical applications, like carrying luggage. My job required frequent travel to see clients, carrying a briefcase laden with 40 to 50 pounds of equity research. Had it not been for yoga, I'm sure my back would never have survived! Many of the guys I worked with complained about injuries or back pain from the weight of the research. I would "sweetly" reply that I had no problems. All the while, yoga was my secret ally!

Because I had so many physical limitations — chronic neck and back pain, sinus problems, knee problems, a lack of flexibility, and no upper body strength — I truly understand what most people need from yoga. *Yoga for Wimps* includes many of the "pre-yoga" exercises I learned during my recovery phase and some that I have developed through my experience in working with "pre-beginner" students. *Yoga for Wimps* meets you, the beginning student, right where you are — with the desire, but without the ability, to do the strenuous poses other yoga books illustrate. It is written with the average person in mind. It is for those who have never tried yoga, and for those who have tried it — and hopelessly given up as they failed in their attempts to place a foot behind their ear!

What *Is* a Wimp?

When I first started doing yoga, my very athletic brother teased me, calling me a wimp. Yet he was unwilling to try even the simplest poses. So I would tease him back, saying he was the wimp and that I was going to write a book just for him — *Yoga for Wimps.* When I first started teaching yoga, I advertised my classes as "Yoga for Wimps" and was astonished by how many people responded to the ads. Everyone I spoke with identified with being a wimp!

My students are all happy to be considered yoga wimps — that way they can "wimp out" of any pose they find too difficult! My students run the gamut of body types and careers. One student is a vegetarian cook. She stands all day and until she started doing yoga, she would leave work with her back howling for a massage. Thanks to yoga, she stopped personally financing a college education for her chiropractor's children. Another student is an economist and a runner. At first he was very, very stiff and had a miserable look on his face as he tried even the simplest stretches. It was obvious that he was there only because he dearly loves his wife and she wanted him to join the class. During his fourth class, I could see he turned the corner — he started to truly enjoy yoga. After class that evening he gave me several suggestions to improve the marketing aspect of my business! Another student is a musician. Until he did yoga, his idea of exercising was letting the cat out the back door. Several students are women in their late 60s and early 70s. They are continually amazed at how much more flexible they are, and how much easier their daily activities — vacuuming, gardening, carrying groceries — have become since they started doing yoga.

When I started writing the book, I puzzled over the definition of a wimp. Then I realized that we are all wimps in some way. We all slam on the snooze bar some mornings when the alarm sounds, hoping to get a few more minutes of sleep instead of getting up to face our day. We all get grumpy when we don't feel good. We all get easily discouraged when something we want to do seems too difficult or time-consuming. We all want to transform our lives — but only if it doesn't take too long!

Yoga for Wimps allows us to "stair-step" our yoga goals. The simple fact is that the great majority of us cannot begin yoga by doing the classic poses. *Yoga for Wimps* presents specific poses to get you going. Immediately you will find that you feel better both physically and spiritually. And soon you will no longer be a Yoga Wimp!

Why Is Everyone Talking About Yoga?

Everyone is talking about yoga. Movie stars, rock stars, and professional athletes are touting yoga as the fountain of youth. Almost every week there is an article about yoga in a prominent periodical. Even business magazines are writing about yoga! Doctors, many of whom have never tried it themselves, are recommending yoga to their patients. Fortune 500 companies are offering lunchtime yoga classes. Catalog sales of yoga accessories are skyrocketing. Yoga is even popular in cyberspace — the Internet has more than 32,000 yoga websites.

So what is it about yoga?

On its most surface level, yoga is a challenging, fun discipline that keeps the body fit. It regulates the internal organs and balances the circulatory, respiratory, and hormonal systems. Yoga alleviates stress, aids in the healing of physical injuries and illnesses, and helps us reclaim our general sense of well-being.

But yoga gives us a sense of well-being that is quite different from the "endorphin high" experienced in Western exercise. As we practice yoga, we sense a mastery of our world. As we practice the strength-building poses we become stronger both physically and mentally. And as we become more flexible in our bodies, we become more flexible in our attitudes.

Practicing yoga also heightens our sense of emotional well-being. Many medical doctors and psychotherapists contend that emotional trauma is not only held in our hearts and minds, but also in our bodies. This must be true, as many yoga students experience emotional release while doing the poses. Some people suddenly remember hurts from long ago and are able to immediately process them. While they are practicing the poses or during the relaxation phase that follows, many students report spontaneous feelings of love or forgiveness; others have profound insights. All students report increased inner peace and relaxation, and it reflects in their faces. One of my teachers in California, Francie Ricks, once said: "Yoga poses are the sacred fires that burn up the neuroses." As we release and heal these pent-up emotions, we allow more space for our true, loving natures to shine forth. In other words, yoga amplifies our sense of inner love, joy, and harmony.

When I started practicing yoga, I was not aware of its spiritual nature. I thought it was just a cool exercise. But my life became much easier. I not only got the job of my dreams but my intuition directed me to the companies I should call for new business. My usual worries were gone. I was more self-reliant, yet felt much more connected to those around me. Through yoga I had tapped into the effortless flow of life that causes the sun to shine and the seasons to change.

I finally linked this new sense of ease and wonderment with yoga when I started reading about yoga. B.K.S. Iyengar states in one of his books that on its highest level, yoga "is the communion of the human soul with Divinity."* And another book, the ancient yoga text called *The Yoga Sutras of Patanjali,* explained my new sense of inner peace with the statement that "yoga quiets the chattering of the mind." When I discussed this concept with a yoga class recently, several students reported that they had not realized how noisy their minds were until they started doing yoga. Most report that their minds do normally quiet down while practicing yoga. However, one student, a French professor, responded that her mind is like an out-of-control day care center. Yoga does help, she said. When she practices yoga the kids stop screaming, but they are still running around!

For those in the latter camp, I am here to report that the mind *will* eventually calm down. When I started doing yoga, my mind was more like an FM radio transmitter, with songs constantly playing in my head. One afternoon as I started the relaxation phase of my yoga practice, there was no mental music! For the first time ever, my mind was absolutely quiet. This scared the daylights out of me and I jumped up wondering who had turned off the radio in my head! I completely ruined my first experience of a quiet mind. Luckily, my mind is not nearly as boisterous as it used to be. And I continue to periodically experience this utter stillness. A few brief moments of complete silence are the world's greatest gifts — better than a two-week vacation!

I have learned firsthand that yoga is a moving meditation. We don't have to force ourselves to sit in uncomfortable positions and chant "Om" or watch our breath or our thoughts. Give me the most difficult yoga poses instead! If our minds are active, then maybe it is a good idea to have active bodies. But let's harness that activity for our highest good, just as we harness the power of a waterfall to generate electricity. Through yoga poses we can reach that same meditative place others are reaching by sitting — and we will have much more fun!

The rewards you reap from practicing yoga will surprise you, far surpassing your most optimistic dreams for physical well-being, joy, and inner peace. Health will replace injury, gratitude will replace worry, self-confidence will replace fear. Your "joie de vivre" will multiply manyfold. All aspects of your life will transform.

That is why everyone is talking about yoga!

I wholeheartedly invite you to take this journey: the vehicle is yoga and the destination is your true self. And you thought you were just going to get a little exercise!

Light on Pranayama, B.K.S. Iyengar, 1987

Getting Started

This book is "user friendly." The three sections are designed to meet your lifestyle. *Instant Yoga* starts with some "Warm-Ups." These are poses that you can do any time of the day or night, before your practice, after your practice, or as you practice. Then, fifteen "practice sessions" are presented. If you have just a short time to practice, open to any page, imitate the photos for the session (you will know when the session ends because the model changes), and you've done your yoga for the day. If you feel energized after doing a certain session, pick another one. You may find that after you have done a few poses, you will naturally want to do more. Allow the natural energy that yoga offers to guide you through your practice. Some days, you will feel as though you just can't get enough yoga. Other days, you may simply want to lie over blankets.

If you are looking for a particular result — to soothe your aching back or neck, or to alleviate stress or fatigue — look in *Fix-Its*. We assume you are motivated to solve your problem, so the instructions are a little more detailed than in *Instant Yoga*.

As you progress and want more information and challenge, check out *The Glossary.* It gives detailed instructions, suggests time periods for holding each pose, and is organized so you can practice each section as a series. If you practice one of the more strenuous sections, be sure to finish with a pose or two from the "Resting Poses" section.

Notice: This is called yoga "practice." And you should consider it just that. You don't have to be perfect, you are simply practicing. There is no competition in yoga — not even with yourself. Yoga is not about how far you can bend over your legs or how long you can hold a pose. It is about working with your body at your own level. So while you will have to make an effort, don't let competitiveness enter your yoga world.

A Few Props You Will Need

- A **chair**. A folding chair or a kitchen ladder-back are best, but use whatever you have.

- Two old **neckties** or belts from your bathrobe.

- Two to three **blankets**, preferably sturdy, but if you only have the soft, squishy kind, use those.

- Two thick **books**, dictionary size or thicker. If you live in a big city, phone books work well.

- Two **face cloths**.

- A small section of **wall** that does not have pictures or where the pictures can be easily removed.

You will use one or all of these props for almost every pose. You may want to have a box for your props so you can access them easily.

Tips for Your Practice

- Move into the poses slowly and deliberately.

- Remember to breathe!

- There are a few directions that I give repeatedly:

  1. *Lengthen your back and lift your sternum.* Your sternum is your breastbone.

  2. *Only bend as far forward as you can with your back straight.* The more you can lift your sternum, the more your upper back will straighten, and the more you can lengthen your back, the straighter your lower back will be. Keeping the back straight strengthens the muscles and allows your posture to improve quickly. If you round your back when it should be straight, you train your spine to curve, which is definitely not the result you are looking for!

  3. *Move from the hip crease.* The hip crease is the hip joint, the place where the front of the hip and the leg meet.

  4. *Straighten your knees and your elbows.* If you can't straighten your knees, try to lengthen your hamstrings (the muscles on the back of the thigh) and lift your quadriceps (the muscles on the front of the

thigh). If your elbows don't straighten, lengthen your arms as much as possible. Work on these things — and remember, you are just practicing!

  5. *Keep your head in line with your spine.* In other words, don't tilt your head backward as you do the poses or you will give yourself a neckache.

  6. *Keep your throat, neck, shoulders, and jaw soft.* Soft means relaxed. Try to be conscious of this; you will feel more relaxed throughout your practice.

- These poses are designed for people with normal limitations. Nonetheless, you should start slowly and not overdo it.

- One side may be more challenging than the other side, so you should do that side twice. Well ... it's a suggestion!

- Loose, comfortable clothing or workout clothes are best for yoga practice.

- Bare feet are essential unless you are in some of the resting poses.

- Some days it will be easy to do yoga; other days it may be tough getting started. But if you do even a little bit of yoga, I guarantee you will be happy you did!

Yoga *for* Wimps

If you have just a short time to practice,

open to any page, imitate the photos for the

session (you will know when the session ends

because the model changes), and you've done

your yoga for the day.

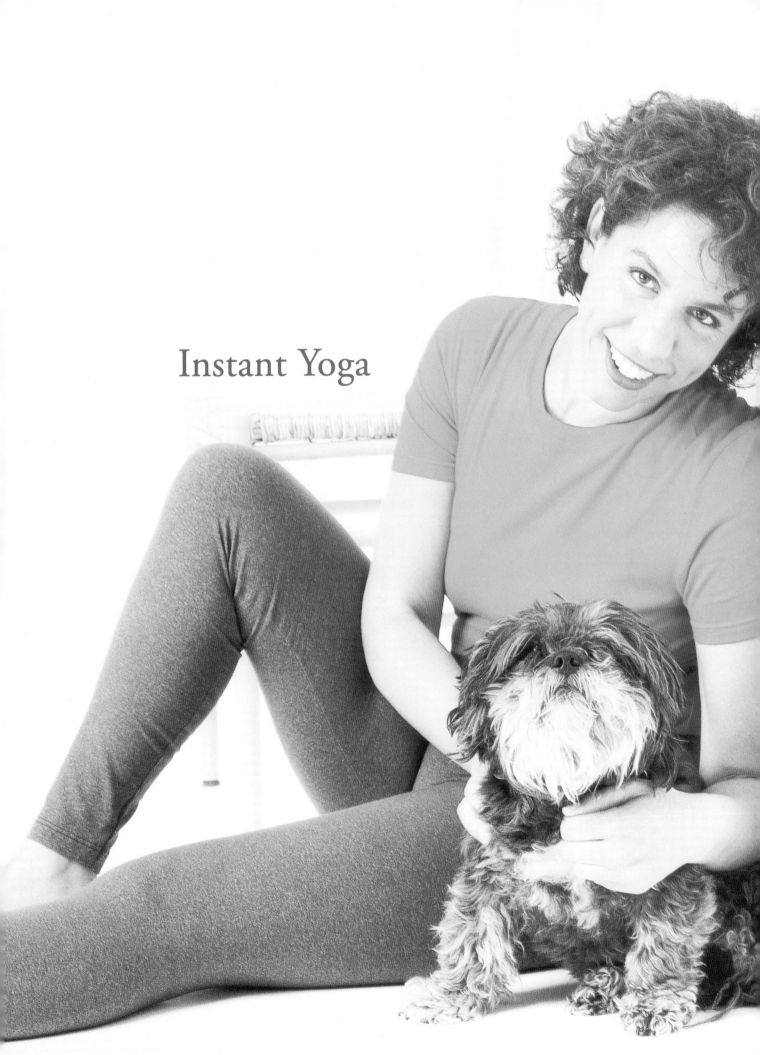

Instant Yoga

Warm-Ups

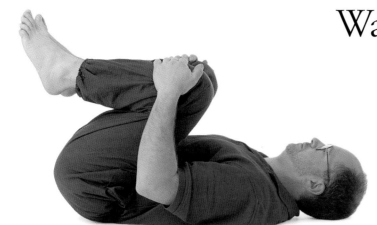

Knees to Chest

- Simply lie on your back, bring your knees to your chest, and hug them.

- And you thought yoga was tough!

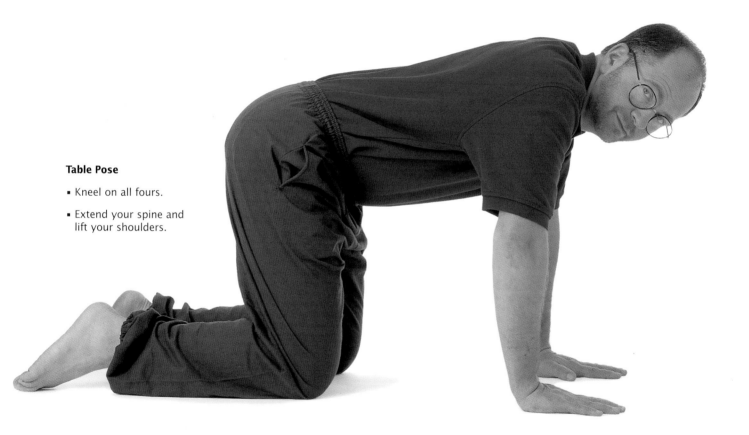

Table Pose

- Kneel on all fours.

- Extend your spine and lift your shoulders.

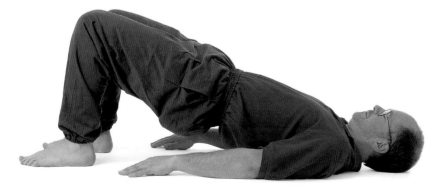

Desk

- Lie on your back, feet hip distance apart and as close to your hips as possible.

- Lift your hips as high as possible and keep them lifted.

- If you can, clasp your hands underneath your back, and roll your shoulders under.

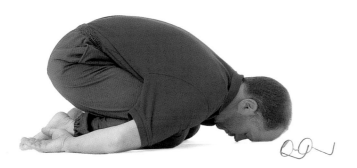

Child's Pose

- From a kneeling position, widen your thighs, place your buttocks on your heels, and bring your torso toward the floor. Rest your forehead on the floor, a book, or a blanket.

- If your body doesn't reach your heels, place a folded blanket or two on your feet.

- Rest with your arms in front of you or beside you.

- Breathe into your lower back and with each exhalation, allow your body to relax a little more.

Chair Lower Back Stretch

- Sit in your chair and widen your legs so they are wider than hip distance apart.

- From the hip crease, bend forward and allow your entire body to relax. Drop your head and completely relax your neck.

- If you are not completely comfortable, try putting a rolled blanket or towel at the hip crease and lean over again.

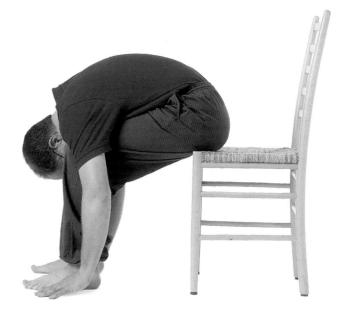

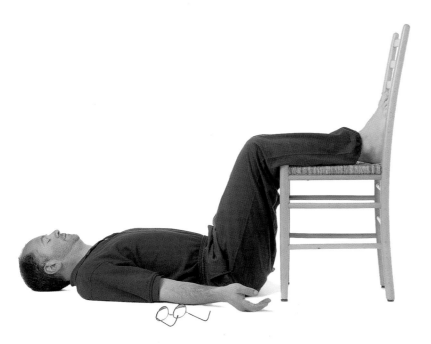

Chair Corpse Pose

- Lie on the floor with your calves on the chair seat.

- Place a pillow or blanket under your head if you like.

- Cover your eyes with a small towel or with your yoga tie and insert earplugs if you wish.

- With each exhalation, relax a little bit more.

Instant Yoga Practice Sessions

Staff Pose

- Lie down with your buttocks at the wall or as close to the wall as possible.

- Extend your legs up the wall. Work on straightening your knees and flexing your feet toward you.

- Easy, right? Well, maybe...

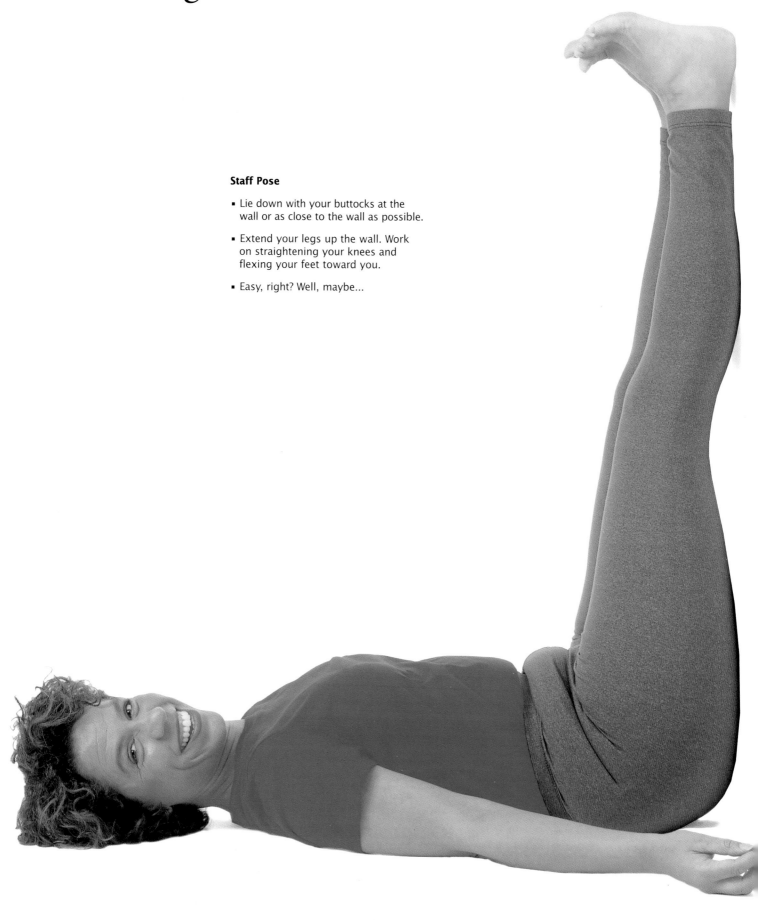

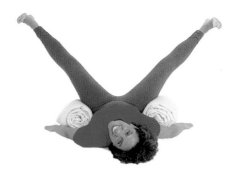

Wide Angle Pose

- From Staff Pose, simply widen your legs. Slowly—you don't want to over-stretch your inner thigh muscles!

- Flex your feet toward you.

- Gravity is your friend. Allow it to bring your legs down as they are ready.

- To take pressure off your inner thighs, roll up blankets and place them under the top of your thighs.

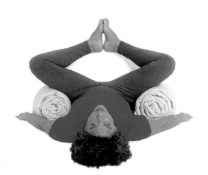

Bound Angle Pose

- Bring the soles of your feet together.

- Firmly press your feet together.

- If you did not use the blanket roll-ups in Wide Angle Pose, you may want to add them here.

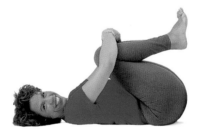

Knees to Chest

- Bring your knees to your chest.

- Have you hugged your knees today?

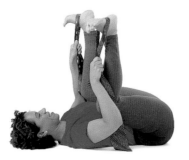

Dead Bug Pose
(I promise you won't get swatted!)

- Bring your thighs to the sides of your torso. Position your feet as if you will walk on the ceiling.

- Place an old necktie around each foot and pull your legs toward you.

- If this is too easy (are you sure you are a Yoga Wimp?), from the inside of the legs, place your hands on the arches of your feet and pull your legs toward you.

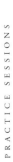

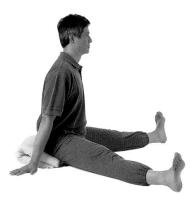

1. Seated Wide Angle Pose

- In this pose and the following four poses, sit on some folded blankets or against a wall to help straighten your back and relieve stiffness in your hips.

- Stretch your legs out to the side.

- Lengthen your back and lift your sternum. Place your hands or fingertips behind you to help lengthen your back.

- Keeping your back straight, bend slightly forward from the hip crease. If you like, you can walk your fingers forward.

Important Note: *Bend forward only to the degree you can keep your back straight. For most of us this is not very far!*

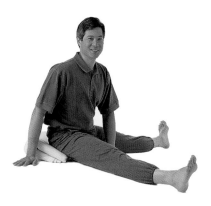

2. Wide Angle Variation

- From the same position, lengthen your back, lift your sternum, and slightly twist your torso toward your right leg.

- From the hip crease, bend over your right leg.

- Once you've gone as far as you can with your back straight, release and switch sides.

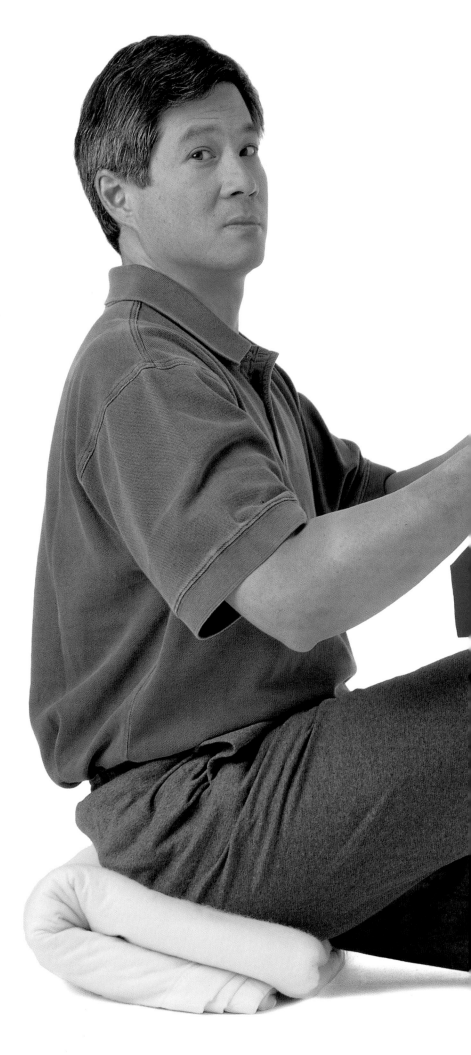

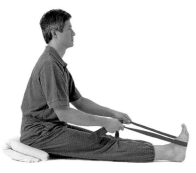

4. Full Forward Bend

- Sitting on folded blankets with your legs extended in front of you and your toes flexed toward you, strap the balls of both feet.

- With your back and knees straight and your sternum lifted, bend forward from the hip crease.

- Go slowly! This is not a contest to see how far down you can get—a long, straight back is most important.

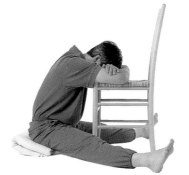

5. Head to Chair Pose

- Sit in any comfortable position in front of the chair.

- Believe it or not, you can round your back in this pose!

- Place your forehead on the chair—or on your hands, forearms, or on books or blankets piled up on the chair, whichever is most comfortable.

- With each exhalation, allow your body and mind to relax just a little bit more.

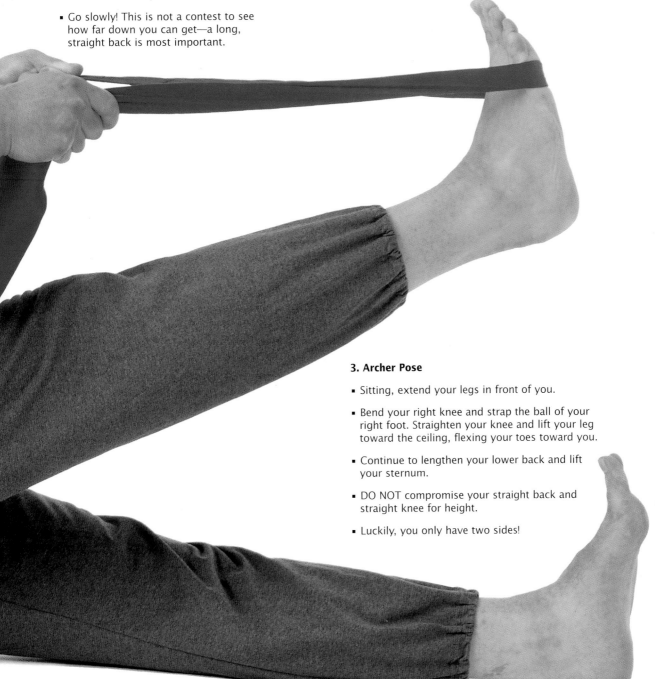

3. Archer Pose

- Sitting, extend your legs in front of you.

- Bend your right knee and strap the ball of your right foot. Straighten your knee and lift your leg toward the ceiling, flexing your toes toward you.

- Continue to lengthen your lower back and lift your sternum.

- DO NOT compromise your straight back and straight knee for height.

- Luckily, you only have two sides!

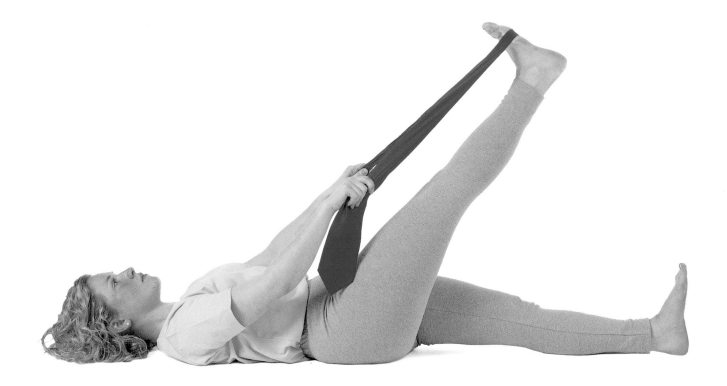

Reclining Hamstring Stretch

- Lie on your back with your legs extended and your feet at the wall.

- Strap the ball of your right foot, lift your leg toward the ceiling and, if possible, straighten your knee. Flex your toes toward you.

- Press the foot of the extended leg into the wall.

- Naturally, you have to do both sides!

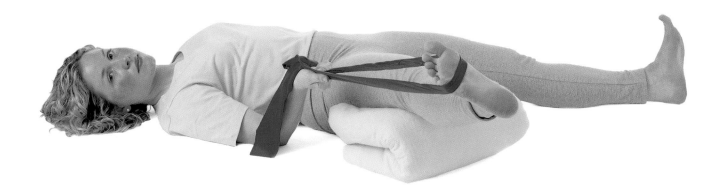

Reclining Inner Thigh Stretch

- Same setup as the previous pose.

- Lift your right leg up and then bring your leg out toward your right shoulder.

- You can stay in this pose longer if you place a folded blanket or a very thick book under your upper thigh.

- Switch sides.

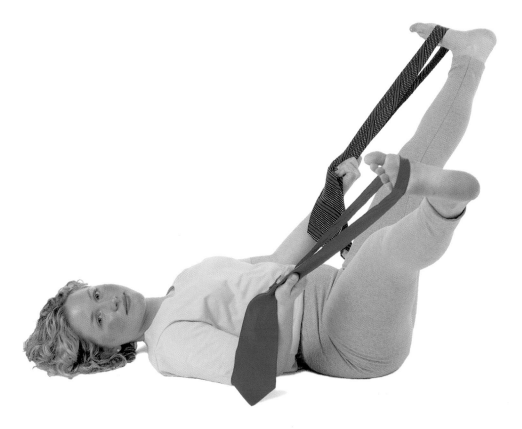

Double Inner Thigh Stretch

- Same setup, but this time bring both legs to the side at the same time.

- Don't forget to double the props.

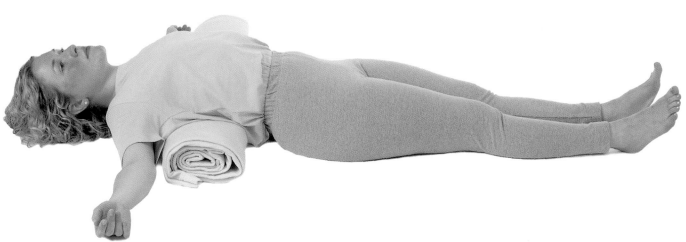

Supported Chest Opener

- Roll up a blanket and lie down over it, placing the roll-up directly behind your sternum.

- You may need to experiment with blanket height to determine what height is most comfortable.

- If you would like, you can also place a pillow or folded blanket under your head.

- Close your eyes and relax.

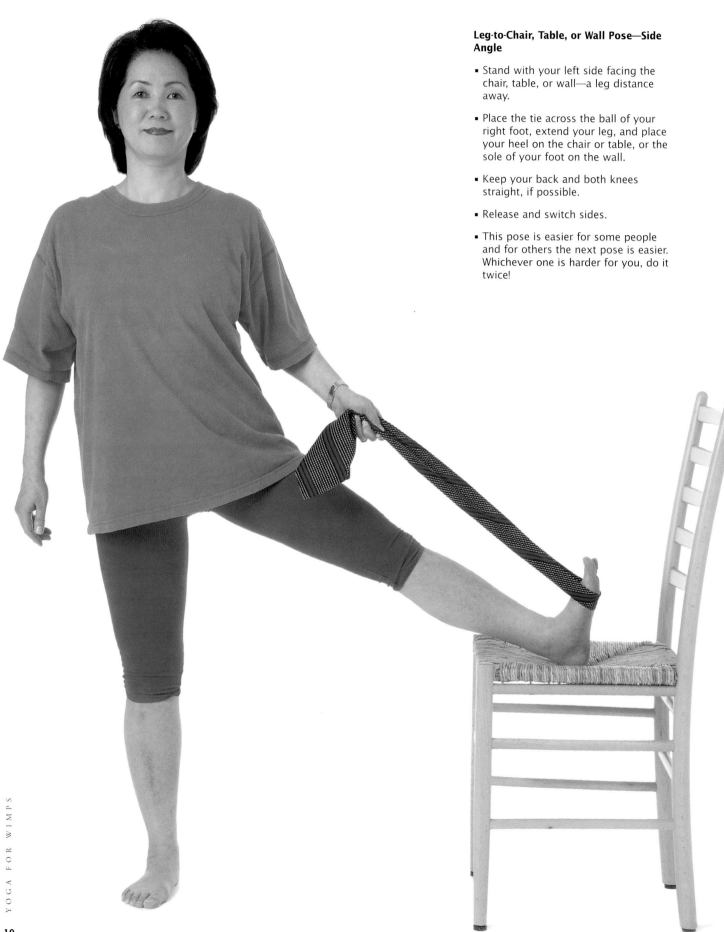

Leg-to-Chair, Table, or Wall Pose—Side Angle

- Stand with your left side facing the chair, table, or wall—a leg distance away.

- Place the tie across the ball of your right foot, extend your leg, and place your heel on the chair or table, or the sole of your foot on the wall.

- Keep your back and both knees straight, if possible.

- Release and switch sides.

- This pose is easier for some people and for others the next pose is easier. Whichever one is harder for you, do it twice!

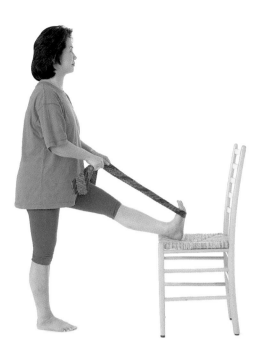

Leg-to-Chair, Table, or Wall Pose—Front Angle

- Stand facing a chair, table, or wall—a leg's distance away.

- Place the tie across the ball of your left foot, extend your leg, and place your heel on the chair or table, or the sole of your foot on the wall.

- Keep your back and both knees straight, if possible.

- Release and switch sides.

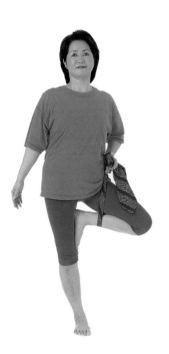

Tree Pose

- Stand with your left side facing the wall, feet together.

- Bend your left leg so your knee touches the wall and your foot is on your inner right thigh.

- Place your tie around your shin if you need help keeping your leg up.

- Press your foot into your thigh and your thigh into your foot.

- Release and switch sides.

- As you progress, you will no longer need the tie or the wall.

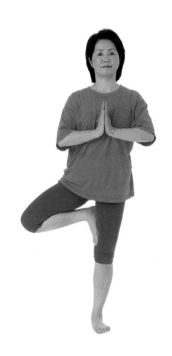

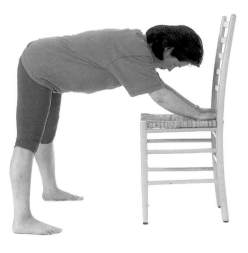

Standing Wide Angle Pose

- Stand about 18 inches from the chair, facing it. Your feet should be 2½ to 3 feet wide.

- Keeping your back and legs straight and your sternum lifted, start to bend toward the chair from your hip crease.

- Place your hands on the chair—either on the seat or on the back.

- Continue to lengthen your back and lift your sternum.

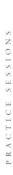

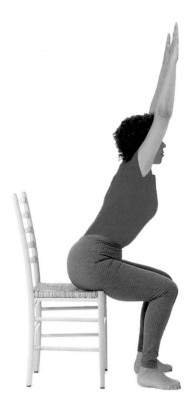

Backward Arm Stretch

- Sit comfortably in front of the chair seat.

- Extend your arms backward and place your hands on the chair seat, sides of the chair, or the chair legs. Experiment to determine which height is best for you.

- Allow your elbows to straighten if possible.

- Lift your chest, roll your shoulders forward, and continue to lift your chest.

- Easier than it looks, right?

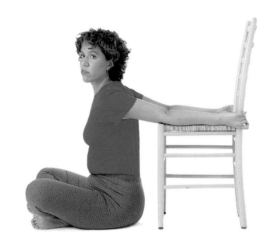

Upward Arm Stretch

- Sit in the chair close to and facing the wall. (Remember this from grade school?)

- Place your hands as high on the wall as possible.

- Walk your fingers higher, stretching all the way from your lower back.

- Let your fingers do the walking up the wall!

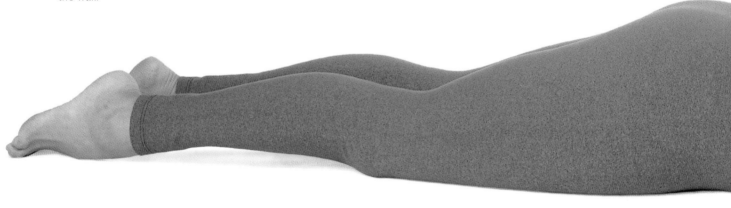

Forward Arm Stretch

- Lie down on your stomach, facing the back of the chair.

- Place your hands as high on the chair as possible — the top, the sides, or the seat.

- Broaden your shoulders by separating your shoulder blades; work on straightening your elbows.

- If this is too easy or your elbows are not straight, scoot your body away from the chair.

- Lift the front legs of the chair, scoot the chair forward a little, and then try to push the front legs down to the floor.

Chair Lower Back Stretch

- Sit in your chair and widen your legs so they are wider than hip distance apart.

- From the hip crease, bend forward and allow your entire body to relax. Drop your head and completely relax your neck.

- If you are not completely comfortable, try putting a rolled blanket or towel at the hip crease and bend forward again.

- With this pose, you will regret that you don't have two sides!

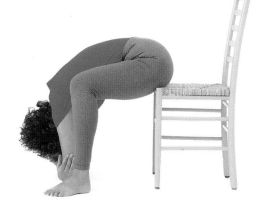

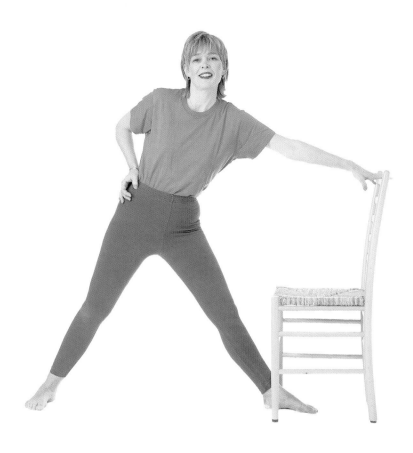

Triangle Pose

- Place the back of the chair against the wall.

- Place your left foot halfway under the chair, toes facing forward.

- The right foot is back 3½ to 4 feet and the heel of the left foot is aligned with the arch of the right foot.

- From the hip crease, laterally extend toward the chair.

- Place your left hand on the back of the chair or on the chair seat. Your right hand is on your hip.

- Breathe!

- Release and switch sides.

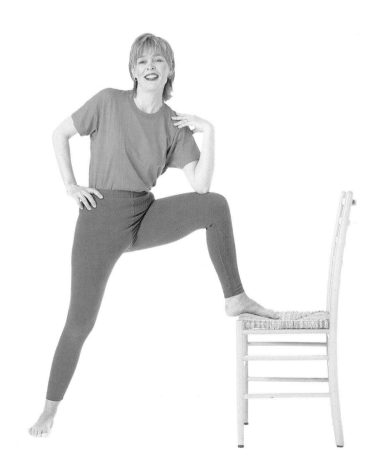

Side Angle Pose

- Start with the same setup as the previous pose, except your forward foot is on the chair seat.

- Bend the forward knee into a right angle.

- Moving from the hip crease, extend your upper body laterally over your thigh.

- Place your left elbow on your knee and your right hand on your hip.

- If this is too easy (and if it is, you are *not* flexibility impaired!), place your forward foot on the floor.

- Release and switch sides.

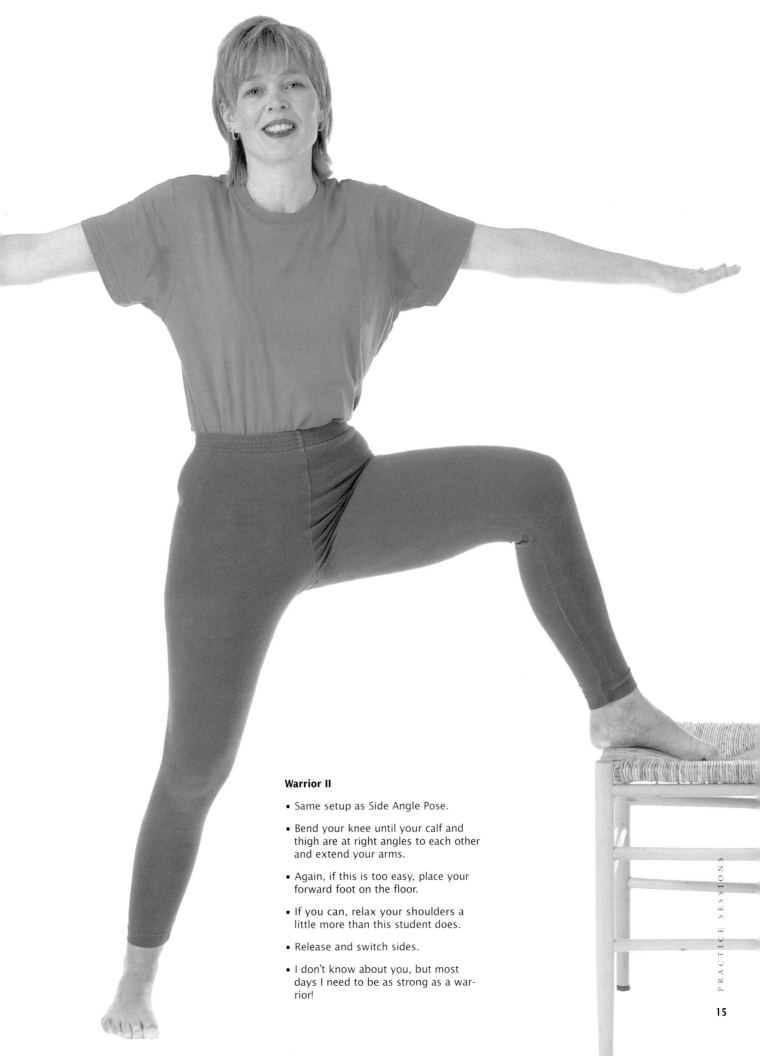

Warrior II

- Same setup as Side Angle Pose.

- Bend your knee until your calf and thigh are at right angles to each other and extend your arms.

- Again, if this is too easy, place your forward foot on the floor.

- If you can, relax your shoulders a little more than this student does.

- Release and switch sides.

- I don't know about you, but most days I need to be as strong as a warrior!

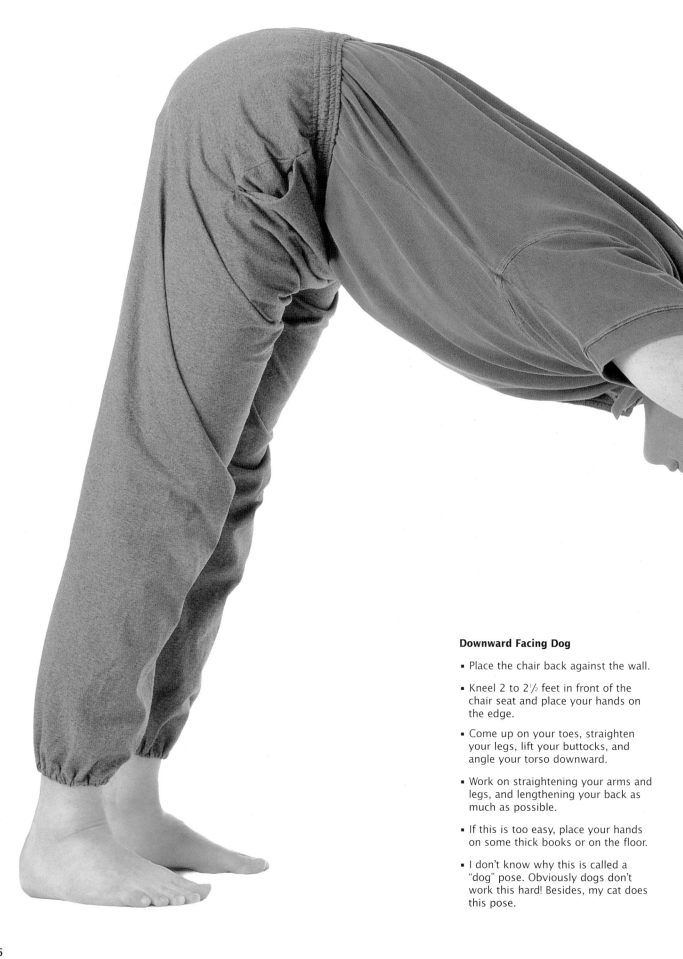

Downward Facing Dog

- Place the chair back against the wall.

- Kneel 2 to 2½ feet in front of the chair seat and place your hands on the edge.

- Come up on your toes, straighten your legs, lift your buttocks, and angle your torso downward.

- Work on straightening your arms and legs, and lengthening your back as much as possible.

- If this is too easy, place your hands on some thick books or on the floor.

- I don't know why this is called a "dog" pose. Obviously dogs don't work this hard! Besides, my cat does this pose.

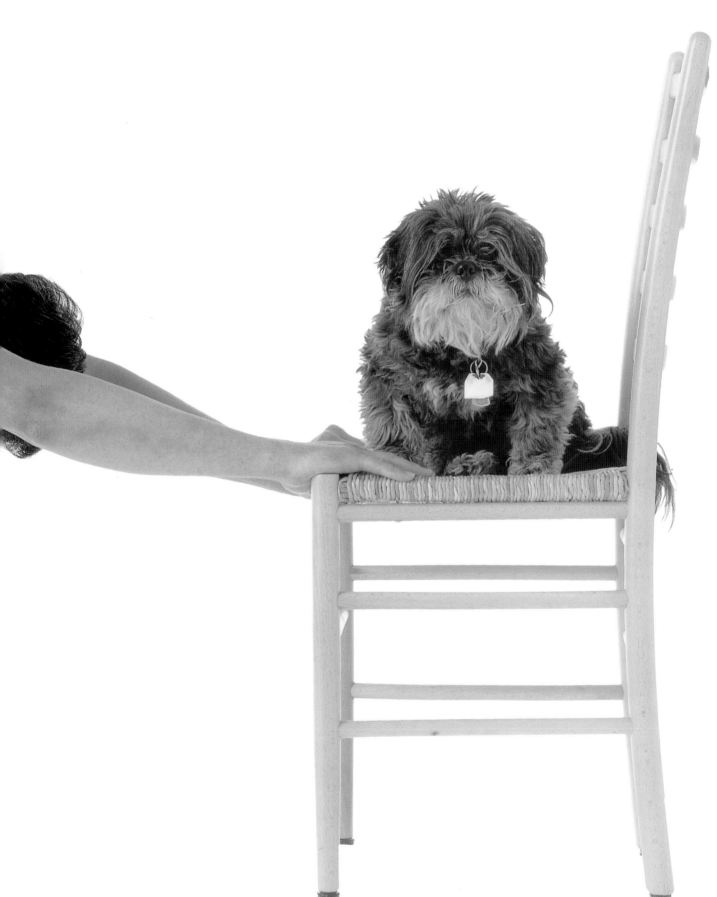

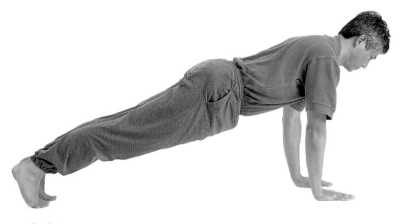

Plank Pose

- Kneel on all fours. Your feet are hip distance apart and on the wall. Your hands are at a 120-degree angle (slightly more than a right angle) to your torso.

- Lift your buttocks so they are in line with your spine, and straighten your arms and legs. Push your feet into the wall. Bring your weight over your arms.

- Draw all of your arm muscles and your shoulders up toward the ceiling.

- If you are feeling strong, you can do some push-ups from this pose. If not, feel free to wimp out of this entire pose!

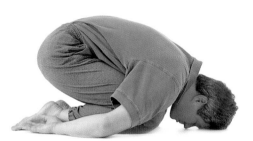

Child's Pose

- From a kneeling position, widen your thighs, place your buttocks on your heels, and bring your torso toward the floor. Rest your forehead on the floor, a book, or a blanket.

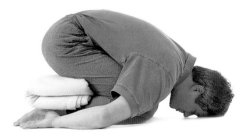

- If your body doesn't reach your heels, place a folded blanket or two on your feet.

- Rest with your arms in front of you or beside you.

- Breathe into your lower back and with each exhalation, allow your body to relax a little more.

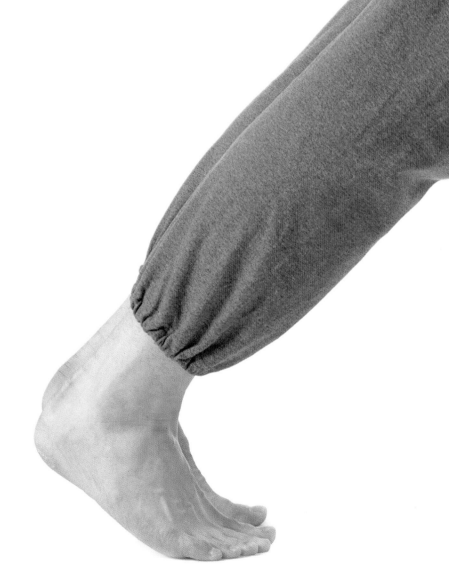

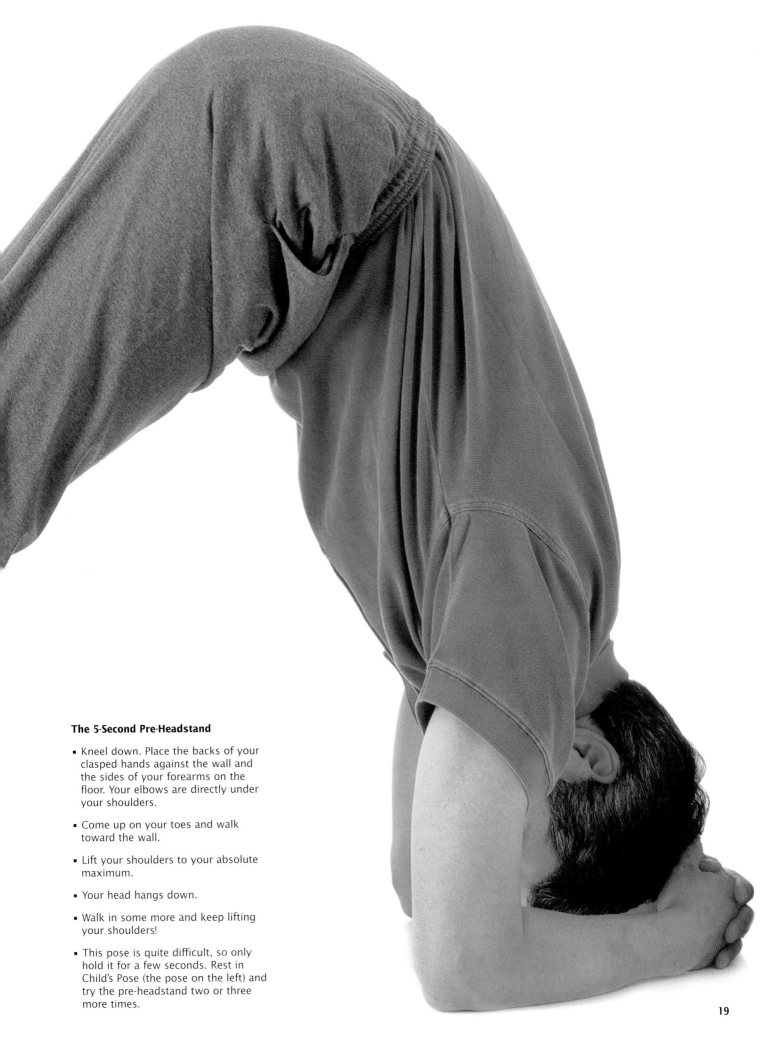

The 5-Second Pre-Headstand

- Kneel down. Place the backs of your clasped hands against the wall and the sides of your forearms on the floor. Your elbows are directly under your shoulders.

- Come up on your toes and walk toward the wall.

- Lift your shoulders to your absolute maximum.

- Your head hangs down.

- Walk in some more and keep lifting your shoulders!

- This pose is quite difficult, so only hold it for a few seconds. Rest in Child's Pose (the pose on the left) and try the pre-headstand two or three more times.

19

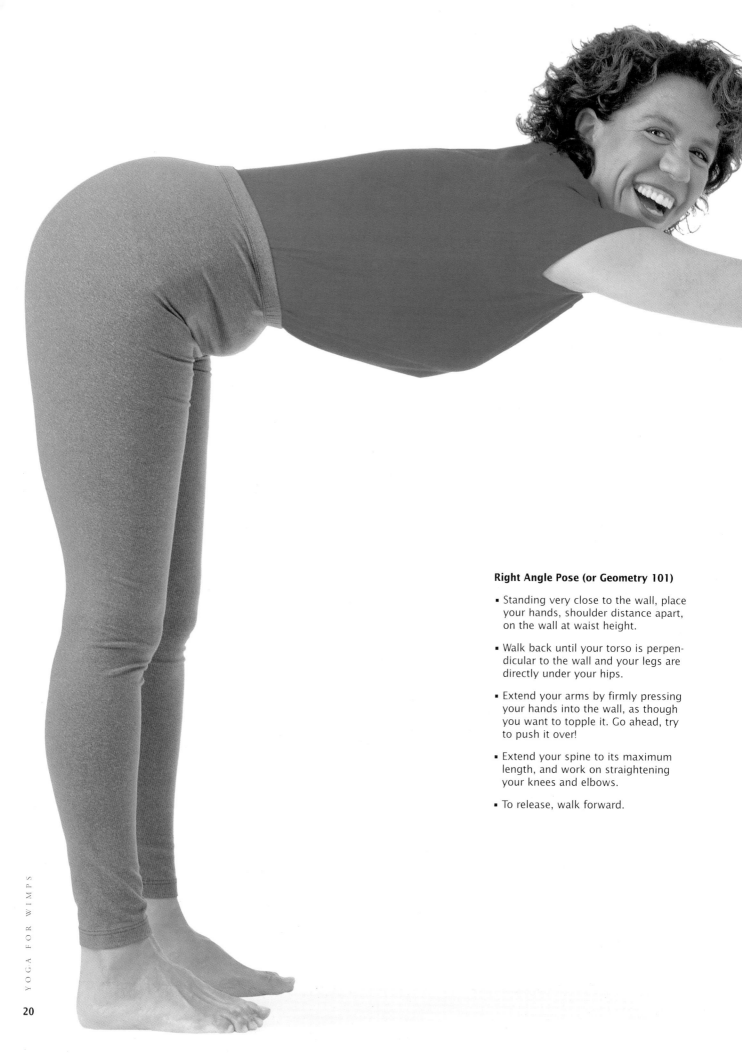

Right Angle Pose (or Geometry 101)

- Standing very close to the wall, place your hands, shoulder distance apart, on the wall at waist height.

- Walk back until your torso is perpendicular to the wall and your legs are directly under your hips.

- Extend your arms by firmly pressing your hands into the wall, as though you want to topple it. Go ahead, try to push it over!

- Extend your spine to its maximum length, and work on straightening your knees and elbows.

- To release, walk forward.

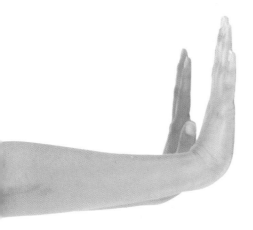

Warrior III

- Return to Right Angle Pose. (Yes, this is a test!)

- Shift your weight to your left leg.

- Now—extend your right leg straight behind you, keeping your leg even with your hips and your front hip-bones even, and flex your toes toward you.

- Bring your leg down, re-establish Right Angle Pose, and then extend your left leg.

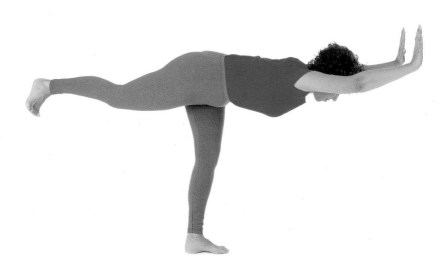

Wall Hang

- Stand with your buttocks at the wall, your feet hip distance apart and about 18 inches from the wall.

- Place your thumbs in your hip crease and bend forward from that crease.

- Release your thumbs and allow your arms to hang down, or hold your elbows. Relax your neck.

- You can bend your knees to get a deeper lower back stretch.

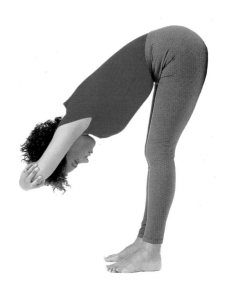

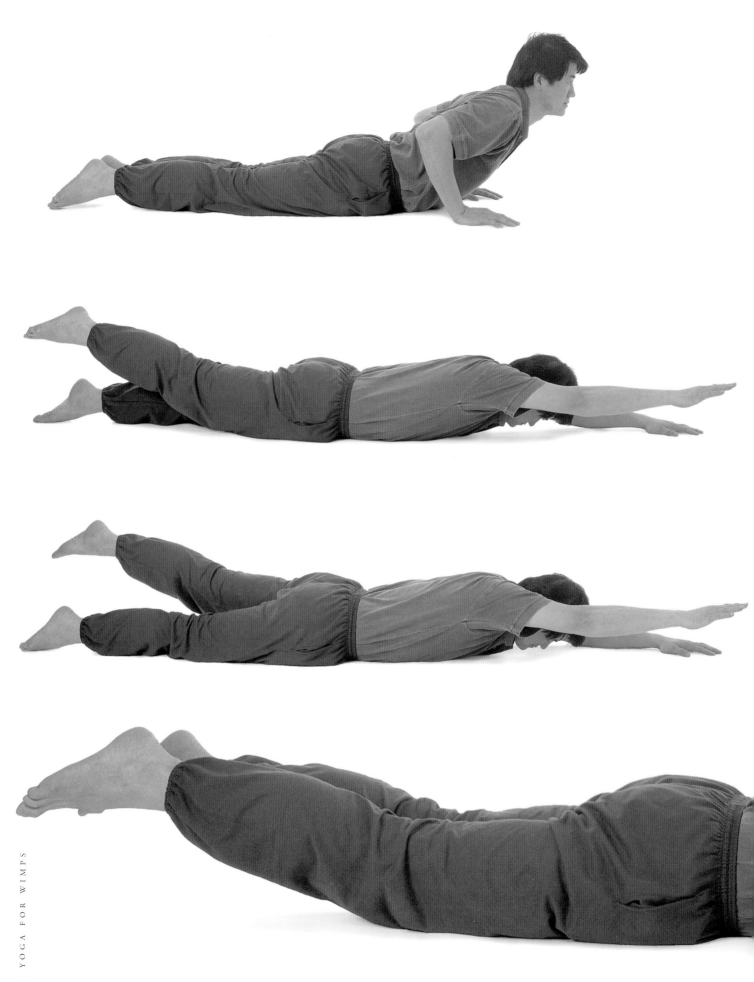

Cobra

- Lie on your stomach and place your hands on the sides of your chest.

- To protect your lower back, firmly press your pubic bone into the floor. Keep your legs straight and firm.

- Raise your chest, curving your upper back inward and extending your chest outward. Lift your sternum.

- Keep your lower rib cage on the floor. Your arms should be at the side of your torso.

- Keep your head in line with your spine. Do not tilt your head backward or you will give yourself a neckache!

Locust Variation 1

- Lie on your stomach with your arms and legs extended.

- To protect your lower back, press your pubic bone into the floor and straighten and firm your legs.

- Lift and extend your right arm and right leg.

- Release, then lift and extend your left arm and left leg.

- Rest and repeat several times.

Locust Variation 2

- Lie on your stomach with your arms and legs extended.

- To protect your lower back, press your pubic bone into the floor and straighten and firm your legs.

- Lift and extend your right arm and left leg.

- Release, then lift and extend your left arm and right leg.

- Rest and repeat several times.

Full Locust

- From the same position, lift both arms and both legs.

- Be sure to press your pubic bone into the floor, and straighten and firm your legs.

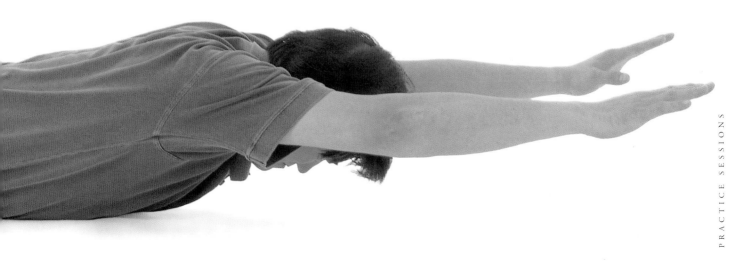

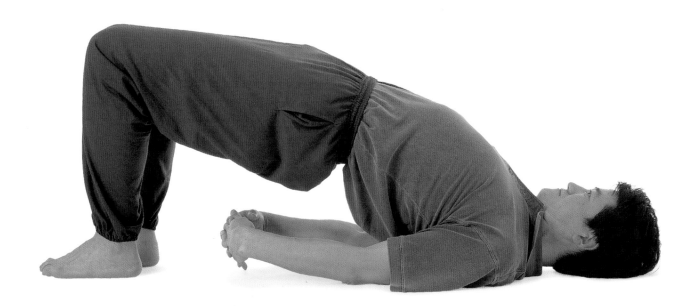

Desk

- Lie on your back with your feet hip distance apart and as close to your hips as possible.

- Lift your hips slightly, clasp your hands underneath your back, and roll your shoulders under.

- Now lift your hips as high as possible and keep them lifted.

- Hold as long as you can. Rest and try again.

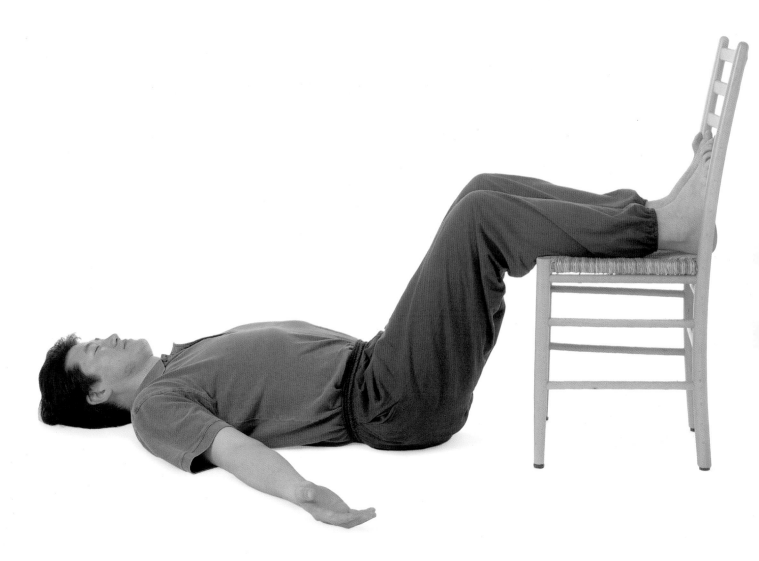

Chair Corpse Pose

- Lie on the floor with your calves on the chair seat.

- Place a pillow or blanket under your head if you like.

- Cover your eyes with a small towel or with your yoga tie and insert earplugs if you wish.

- With each exhalation, relax a little bit more.

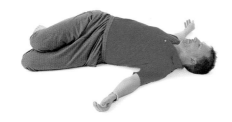

1. Feet on the Floor Twist

- Lie on your back, legs bent, feet together and on the floor, and arms extended to your side.

- Keeping your legs together, bring them to the right side.

- Come back to center and twist to the left.

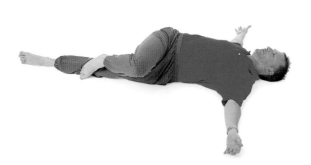

2. Foot on Knee Twist

- Lie on your back with your legs straight, toes flexed toward you, and arms extended to each side.

- Place your right foot on your left knee.

- Turn toward the right, moving your knee toward the floor—not necessarily *to* the floor. Keep your left shoulder on the floor.

- Come back to center and change sides.

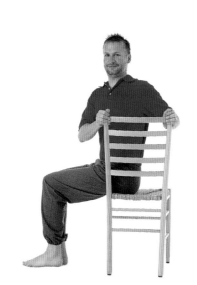

3. Chair Twist 1

- Sit on the *edge* of your chair sideways with your left side facing the chair back.

- Keep your feet and knees together and even throughout the pose.

- Place your hands on the chair as shown.

- On an inhalation straighten your spine and on an exhalation twist toward the chair, twisting from the very bottom of your spine—pushing with your left hand and pulling with your right hand.

- Repeat the inhalation/straighten, exhalation/twist series several times.

- Release and switch sides.

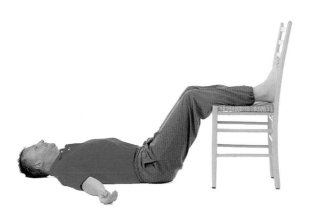

5. Chair Corpse Pose

- Lie on the floor with your calves on the chair seat.

- Place a pillow or blanket under your head if you like.

- Cover your eyes with a small towel or with your yoga tie and insert earplugs if you wish.

- With each exhalation, relax a little bit more.

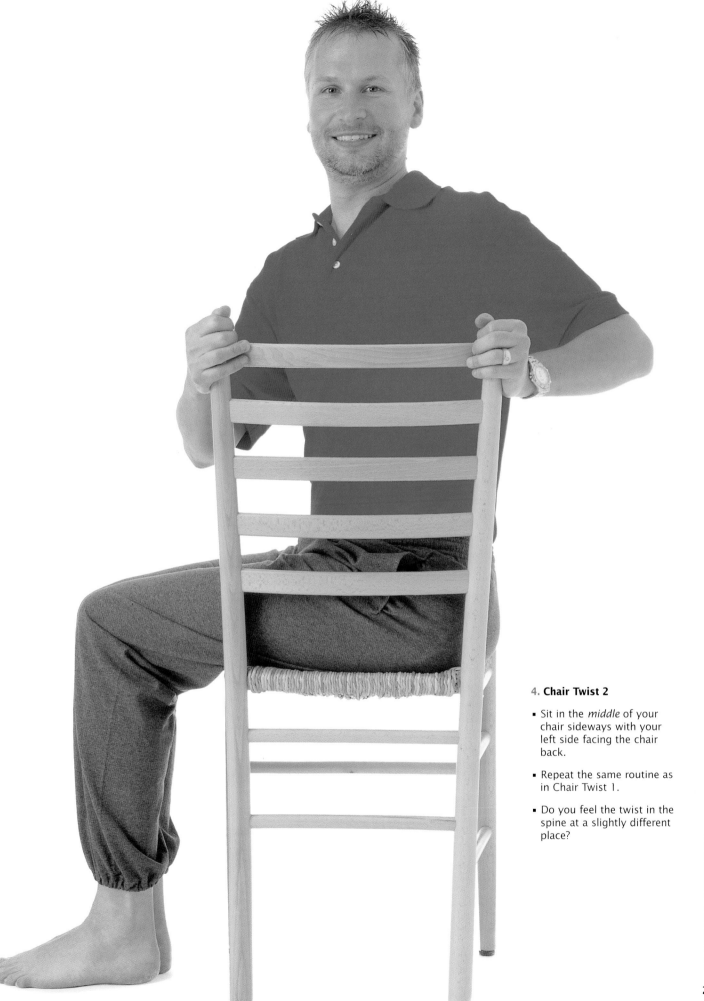

4. Chair Twist 2

- Sit in the *middle* of your chair sideways with your left side facing the chair back.

- Repeat the same routine as in Chair Twist 1.

- Do you feel the twist in the spine at a slightly different place?

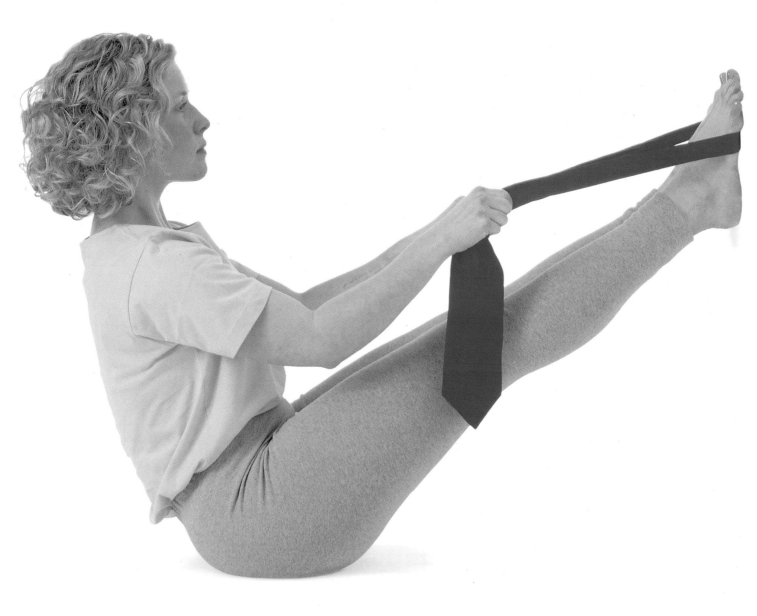

Boat with Strap

- Place a tie around the balls of your feet and place your feet on the wall about 2 feet from the floor.

- Lean back slightly so your torso forms a "V" with your legs.

- Lengthen your back, lift your sternum, squeeze your thighs together, and press your feet into the wall.

- If this is too easy, do the pose without the wall, firmly pressing your feet into the tie.

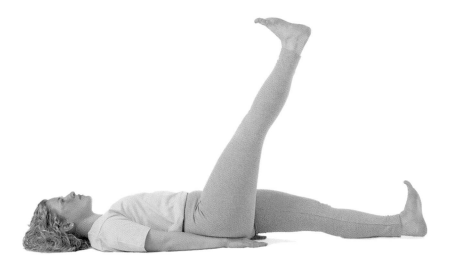

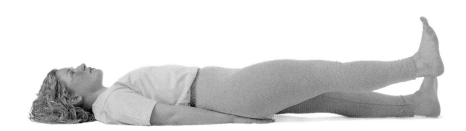

Leg Lifts

- Lie on your back with your left and right legs straight.

- Raise your right leg and then slowly lower it toward the floor.

- Continue several times and then switch sides.

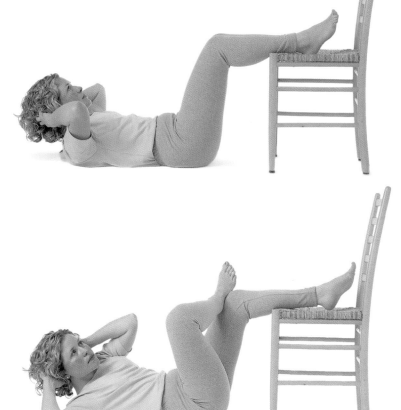

Yoga Sit-Ups

- Lie on your back. With your knees bent, place your feet, hip distance apart, on the chair.

- Place your hands behind your head and try to touch your knees with your elbows — more than once!

- Only bring your back halfway to the floor after touching your elbows to your knees.

Yoga Sit-Ups 2

- From the previous position, bring your right foot to your left knee.

- Sit up and try to touch your right knee with your left elbow — several times.

- Switch the foot position, bringing the right elbow to the left knee.

- Only bring your back halfway to the floor after touching your elbow to your knee.

- Are you breathing?

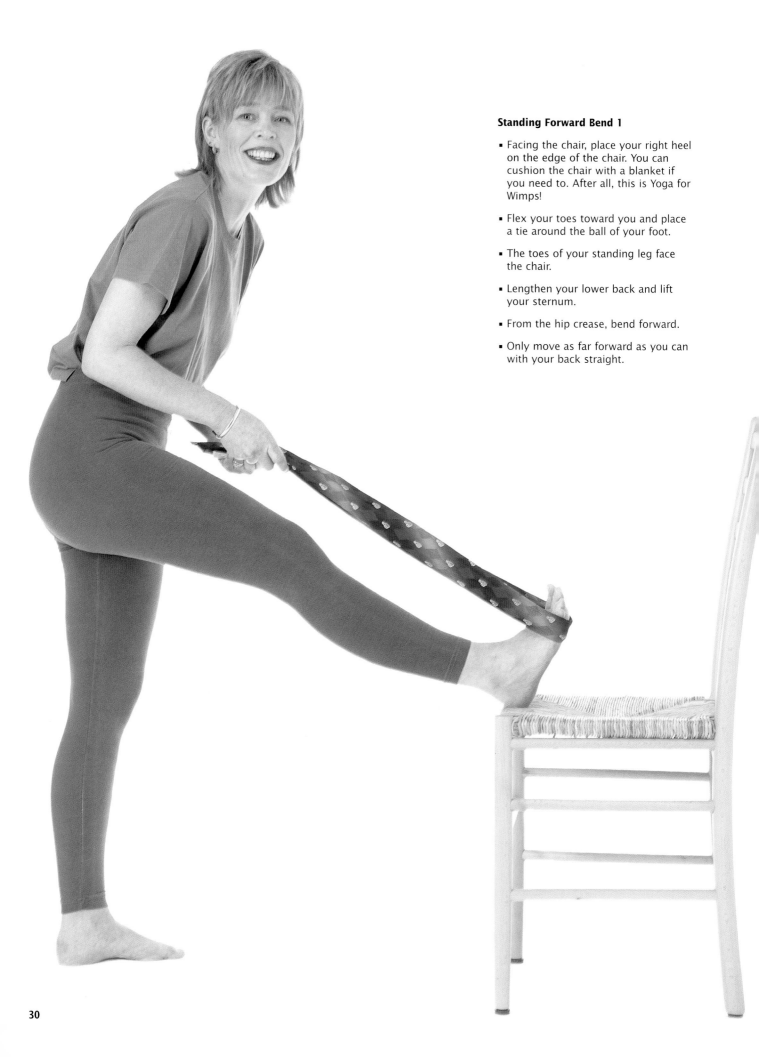

Standing Forward Bend 1

- Facing the chair, place your right heel on the edge of the chair. You can cushion the chair with a blanket if you need to. After all, this is Yoga for Wimps!

- Flex your toes toward you and place a tie around the ball of your foot.

- The toes of your standing leg face the chair.

- Lengthen your lower back and lift your sternum.

- From the hip crease, bend forward.

- Only move as far forward as you can with your back straight.

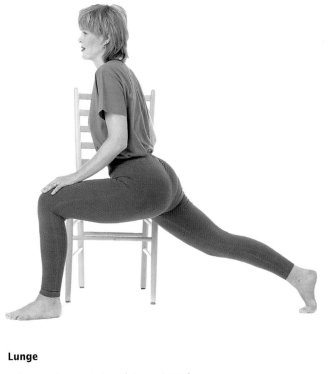

Quadriceps Stretch

- Kneel with the sole of your right foot at the wall.

- Bring your left leg forward so your calf and thigh form a slightly obtuse angle. Hold onto the chair for support if necessary.

- Your right knee is on the floor and your right foot is pressing into the wall. Keeping your torso erect, start to sink your hips toward the floor.

- If you want more challenge, bring your hands to the floor. Keep pressing your heel toward the wall.

- Your left side will feel awfully lonely if you don't do both sides!

Lunge

- Same setup as in Quadriceps Stretch.

- This time, lift your knee off the floor and straighten it.

- If you can (but it isn't necessary), sink your hips a little more than this student does. Keep pressing your foot into the wall to help keep your knee straight.

- Release and switch sides.

Standing Hamstring Stretch

- Place your left foot halfway under the chair and your right foot 3 to 3^1/$_2$ feet back from your left foot.

- Lengthen your lower back and lift your sternum.

- From the hip crease, bend toward the chair.

- Place your hands on the chair back or chair seat and continue to elongate your back. As you progress, you will be able to place your forearms on the chair seat and maintain a straight back.

- Release and switch sides.

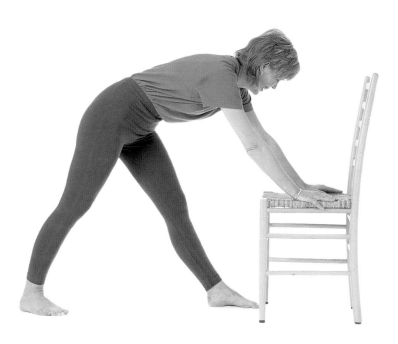

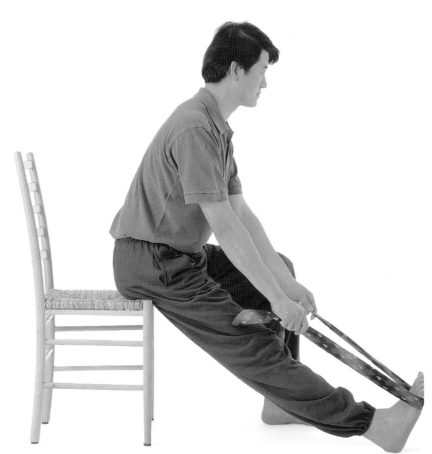

Seated Hamstring Stretch

- Sit near the edge of the chair, facing the wall.

- Place your right foot on the floor at the wall, knee straight, and bend your left leg normally.

- Either place a tie around the ball of your right foot or hold onto the sides of the chair.

- Lengthen your back, lift your sternum, and relax, or soften, your throat, neck, and shoulders.

- Bend slightly forward from the hip crease, keeping your back elongated (this means do not round your back!).

- Make sure you do both sides!

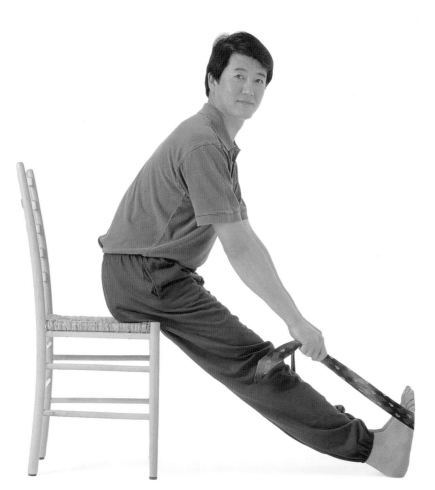

Seated Double Hamstring Stretch

- Sit near the edge of the chair and place your feet on the wall. Place a tie around the balls of your feet.

- Lengthen your back and lift your sternum. From the hip crease, lean forward.

- Only go as far forward as you can and keep your back and knees straight.

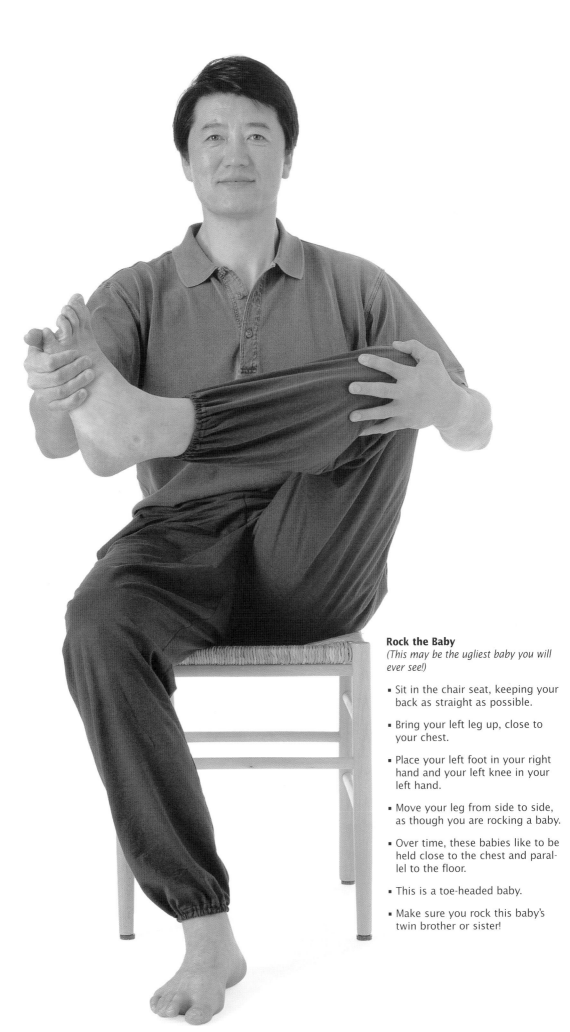

Rock the Baby
(This may be the ugliest baby you will ever see!)

- Sit in the chair seat, keeping your back as straight as possible.

- Bring your left leg up, close to your chest.

- Place your left foot in your right hand and your left knee in your left hand.

- Move your leg from side to side, as though you are rocking a baby.

- Over time, these babies like to be held close to the chest and parallel to the floor.

- This is a toe-headed baby.

- Make sure you rock this baby's twin brother or sister!

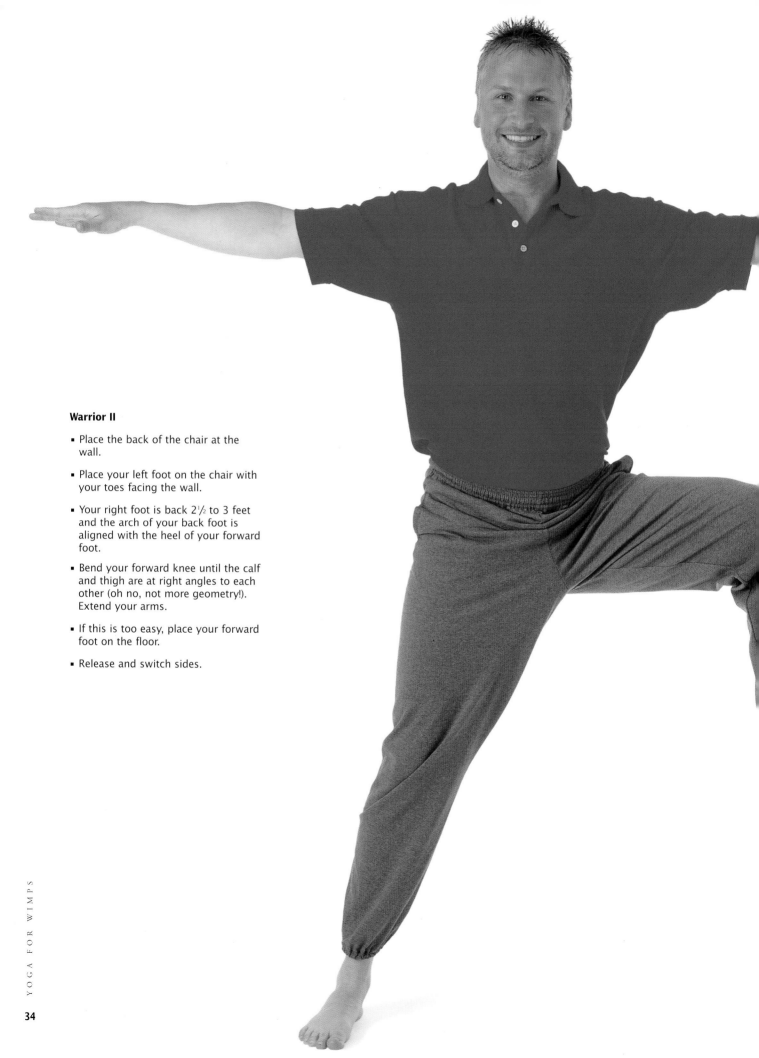

Warrior II

- Place the back of the chair at the wall.

- Place your left foot on the chair with your toes facing the wall.

- Your right foot is back $2\frac{1}{2}$ to 3 feet and the arch of your back foot is aligned with the heel of your forward foot.

- Bend your forward knee until the calf and thigh are at right angles to each other (oh no, not more geometry!). Extend your arms.

- If this is too easy, place your forward foot on the floor.

- Release and switch sides.

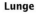

Lunge

- Kneel with the soles of your feet at the wall.

- Bring your left leg forward so your calf and thigh form a slightly obtuse angle. Hold onto the chair for support if necessary.

- Your right knee is on the floor and your right foot is pressing into the wall. Keeping your torso erect, start to sink your hips toward the floor.

- Now straighten (or at least try to straighten) your back leg.

- If you want more challenge, bring your hands to the floor. Keep pressing your heel toward the wall.

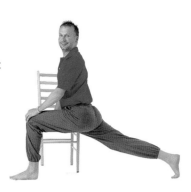

Warrior I

- Place your left foot at the wall and your right leg back about 3 feet, heel up.

- With your hands on the wall and your front hipbones even, start to slowly bend your left knee.

- Eventually, your left knee will bend into a right angle, but there is no hurry to get there.

- Release and switch sides.

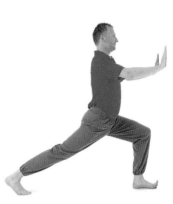

Standing Forward Bend 2

- Stand with your left side facing the chair. Place your left foot on the chair seat, bending the knee. Make sure your left foot is aligned with the right foot, which is about 12 inches from the chair seat.

- From the hip crease, bend forward.

- Hold onto your elbows and allow your head to hang down.

- Release and switch sides.

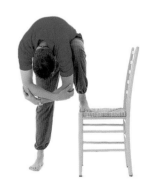

Chair Corpse Pose

- Lie on the floor with your calves on the chair seat.

- Place a pillow or blanket under your head if you like.

- Cover your eyes with a small towel or with your yoga tie and insert earplugs if you wish.

- With each exhalation, relax a little bit more.

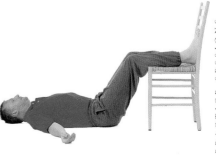

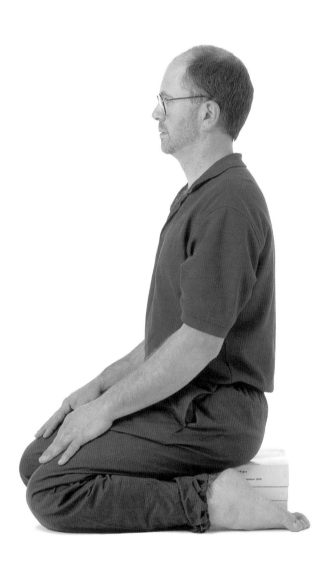

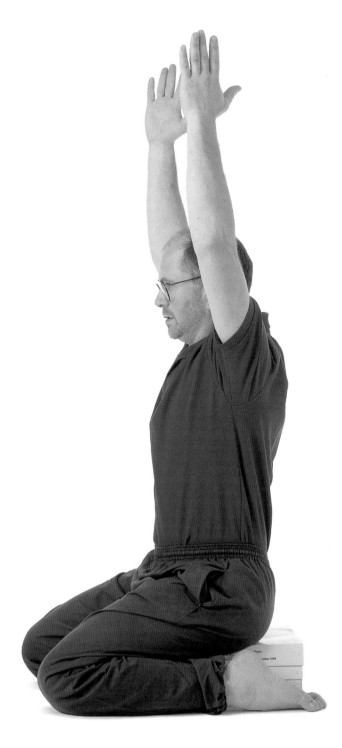

Hero Pose

- Place a thick book on the floor.

- Kneel, with your knees hip distance apart, in front of the book.

- Roll your calves outward and sit on the book.

- If you are immediately uncomfortable, come up and add another book. Determine if you still need another book.

- If your ankles are unhappy, roll up some small face towels and place them under your ankles. You may have to experiment with the thickness of the rolls.

- Eventually, your props will become lower and your knees will come together.

Arm Variations 1

- Stretch your arms straight overhead, palms facing each other.

- Lengthen your arms as though you are stretching all the way from your hips.

- Lift your sternum, but relax your throat, neck, and shoulders, and keep reaching for the ceiling.

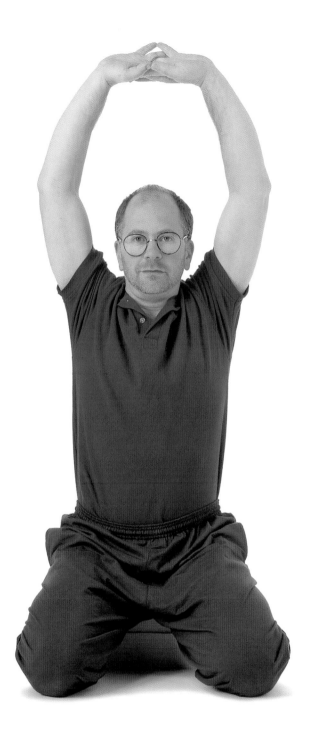

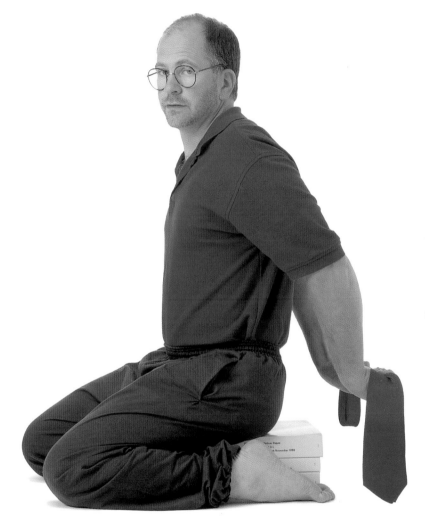

Arm Variations 2

- Interlock your fingers, then face your palms outward.

- Stretch your arms overhead, so your palms face upward.

- Work on straightening your elbows and on stretching all the way from the waist.

- Relax your throat, neck, and shoulders as you try to lift higher.

Arm Variations 3

- Bring your arms behind your back, holding a tie between your hands.

- Lift your arms as high as you can. Keep lifting your sternum.

- As you gain flexibility, bring your hands closer together on the tie. Or forget the tie and interlock your fingers.

If you are looking for a particular result —

to soothe your aching back or neck, or to

alleviate stress or fatigue — look in here.

We assume you are motivated to solve your

problem, so the instructions are a little more

detailed than in Instant Yoga.

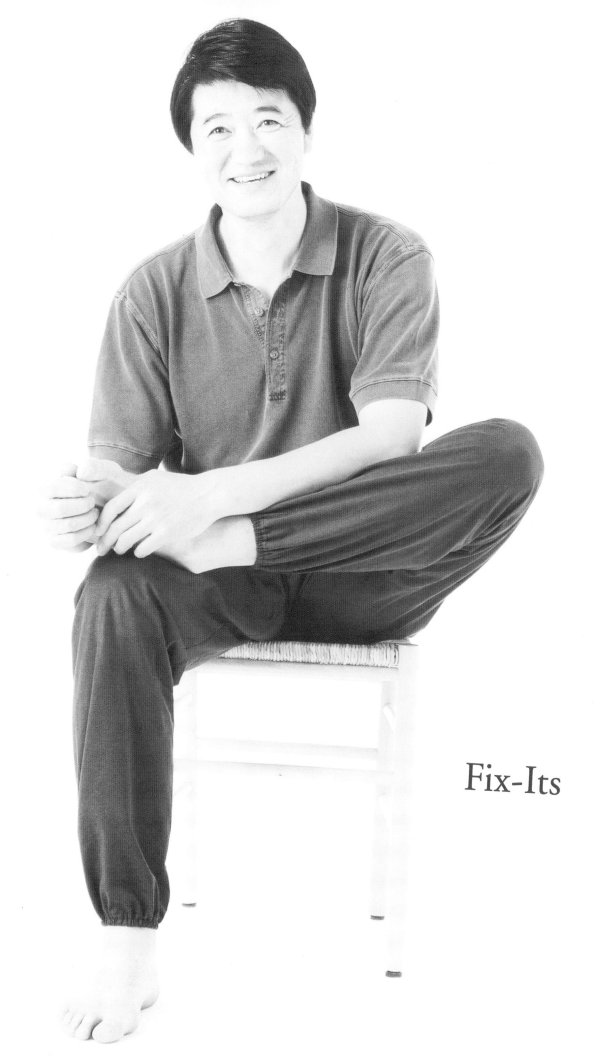

Fix-Its

The Cure for Museum-itis, or Shopping Without Dropping

We have all experienced the inevitable fatigue associated with an afternoon at the museum. We want to see all of the art and all of the treasures, but after a while, our backs, legs, and feet ache so much we are no longer awed by the 3rd Century BC sculptures. Or shopping! We do not want to leave the mall until every store has been surveyed. Instead of pushing on and later becoming a complete grump, or abandoning the museum or the mall for an ice-cream parlor, use a few of these yoga tricks to put the fun back in the afternoon and allow yourself to enjoy several more hours of your favorite passion.

The only prop you will need is a bench — and all malls and museums have benches. You can do the Arm Extensions while walking around, but you may have to set aside your packages for a bit. Do not become intimidated by the other museum-philes or shoppers. If they had any idea how good you are going to feel in a few minutes, they would join you!

Bench Forward Bend

- Sit on the edge of the bench, legs extended forward.

- From the hip crease, lean forward over your legs.

- Keep your knees straight, if you can.

- If you have a sweater, jacket, or package, place it at the point on your legs where your forehead would fall if you were that flexible. Now you can bend your knees and round your back. Place your forehead on the prop and allow your body to melt into the pose.

- Stay in this position as long as you like. Or release the pose and go back into it several times.

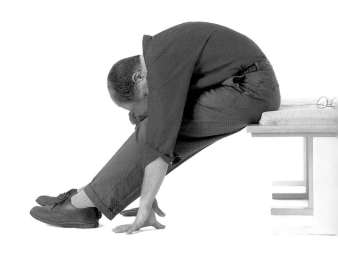

Lower Back Stretch

- Hopefully, if you are female, you will have on pants or a very long skirt. For men, there is no problem unless you are wearing a kilt!

- Sit on the edge of the bench, separate your legs so they are wider than hip width apart, and from the hip crease, bend forward. Hold your elbows or rest your hands on the floor.

- Allow your body, especially your neck and head, to completely hang, in a relaxed, "rag-doll" fashion.

- Take long deep breaths, as though your inhalations were going to the very bottom of your back.

- After a few moments, release, relax, and try again.

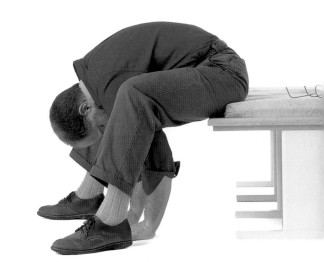

Standing Forward Bend with Bench

- Stand with your left side facing the chair. Place your left foot on the bench, bending your knee. Make sure your left foot is aligned with your right foot, which should be about 12 inches from the bench.

- From the hip crease, bend forward.

- Hold onto your elbows or pull yourself deeper into the pose using the edge of the bench or the bench legs.

- Allow your head to hang down.

- Release and switch sides.

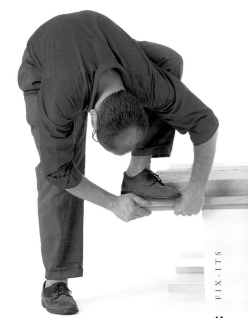

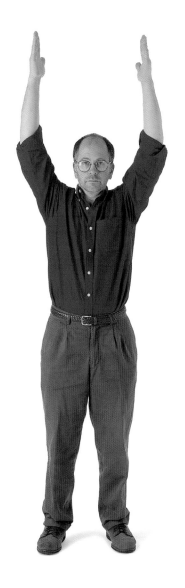

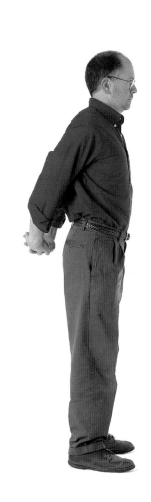

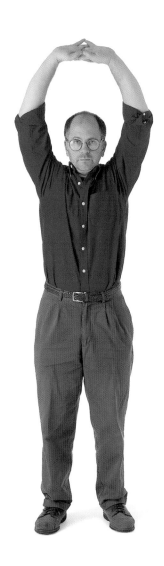

Arm Stretch 1

- Stretch your arms straight overhead, palms facing each other. Stretch from the lower torso, not just from the shoulders. Be sure to keep your neck and shoulders relaxed as you do this.

- Release and repeat several times.

Arm Stretch 2

- Bring your arms behind your back, clasping your hands. Or, hold a tie, sweater, or scarf (or something) between your hands.

- Lift your arms as high as you can. Lift your sternum.

Arm Stretch 3

- Interlock your fingers and extend your arms outward, straight in front of your shoulders.

- Slowly raise your hands overhead, stretching all the way from the waist.

- Work on straightening your elbows.

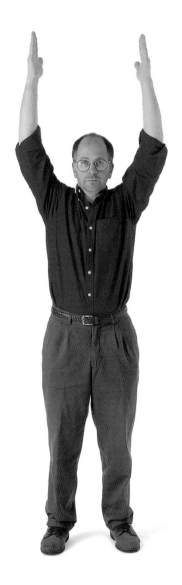
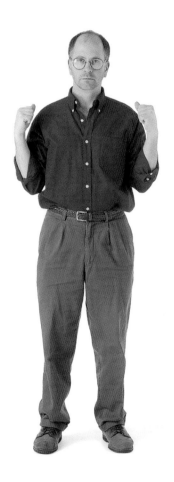

The Best Arm Extensions

- Extend your arms over your head, inhaling deeply as you do this.

- When you have reached your full extension, make a fist. Exhale quickly, bend your elbows, and bring your arms down so that the inside of your upper arms touch the sides of your chest and your fists are shoulder height.

- Tip: take deep, exaggerated breaths, and exhale forcefully. Be sure your neck is relaxed. Do this 8 or 10 times, rest, and repeat once or twice more.

- This is a particularly powerful technique and it is sure to reinvigorate you!

- You can also try this at work instead of an afternoon coffee break.

The Lower Back Blues

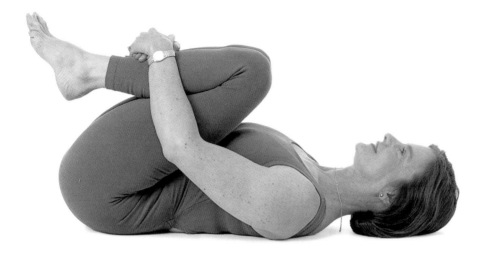

Knees to Chest

- Lie on your back, bring your knees into your chest, and hug them.

- Breathe deeply into your lower back and with each exhalation, allow your entire back to relax just a little bit more.

Chair Lower Back Stretch

- Sit in your chair and widen your legs so they are wider than hip distance apart.

- From the hip crease, bend forward and allow your entire body to relax. Drop your head and completely relax your neck.

- If you are not completely comfortable, try putting a rolled blanket or towel at the hip crease and lean over again.

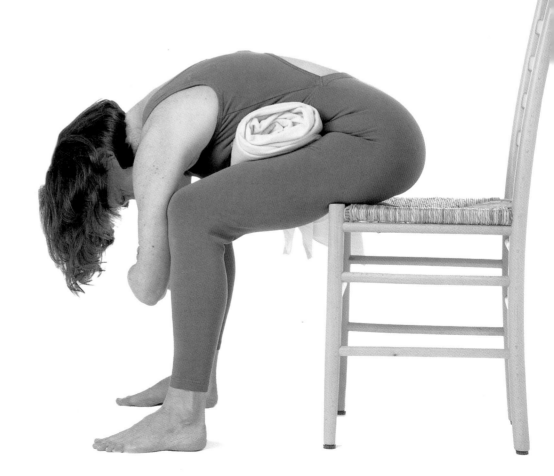

Too many hours at the computer? Or is it that awful road trip that results in a throbbing back? Standing all day at your job? Whatever the "too much of" is that stresses your back, try this series of poses and see how much better you will feel within minutes!

Cross-Legged Lower Back Stretch

- Sit a few inches from the wall with your legs crossed.

- Walk your fingers up the wall, stretching from the lower back.

- Broaden your shoulders by separating and lifting your shoulder blades. Keep your throat and neck soft. Don't tense your shoulders, just lift them.

- When you think you have gone as high as you can, rest for a moment while your body adjusts to the pose, then walk your fingers a little higher.

- Rest and repeat several times.

- If this is too difficult try the next pose.

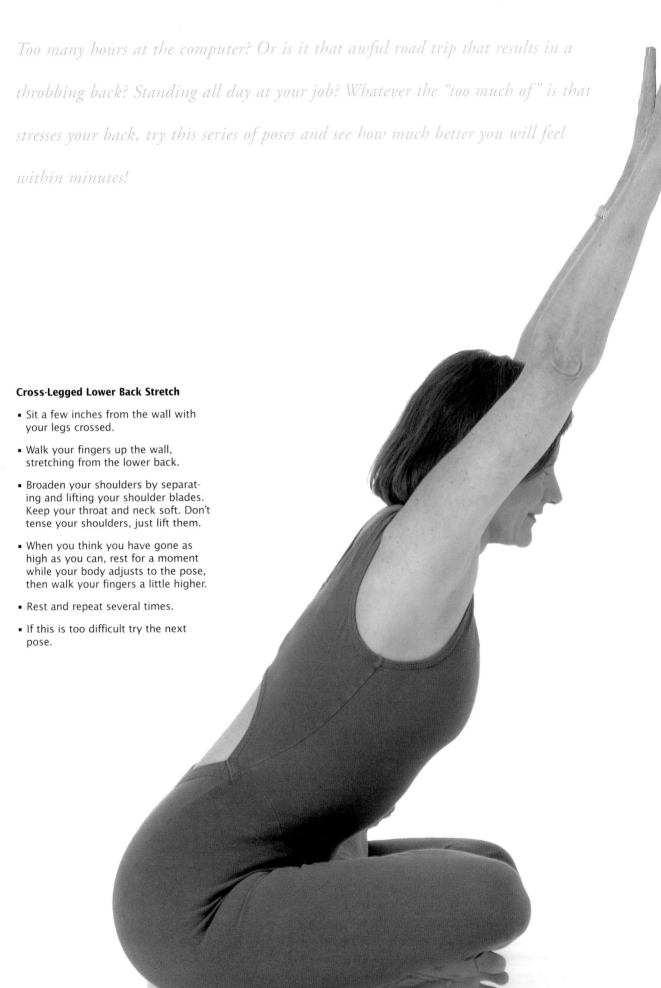

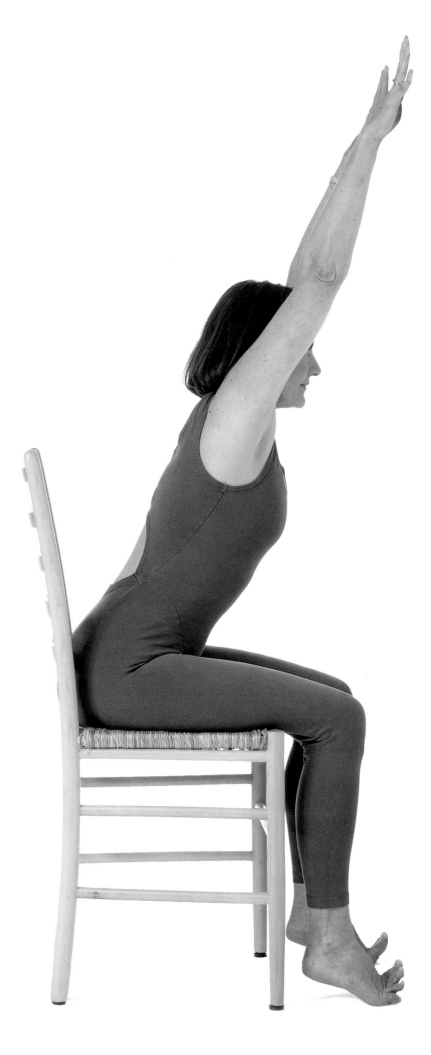

Upward Arm Stretch

- Sit in the chair facing the wall.

- Place your hands as high on the wall as possible and walk your fingers higher up the wall, stretching from your lower back.

- Broaden your shoulders by separating and lifting your shoulder blades. Keep your throat and neck soft. Don't tense your shoulders, just lift them.

- Once you think your fingers are as high as they can be, rest for a moment in the position so your body can adjust, and then walk your fingers higher.

- Rest and repeat several times.

Kitchen Counter Pose

- Fold or roll up some blankets or towels and place them on the kitchen counter.

- If your counter is high or you are short, stand on thick books, as shown. Or you can place your roll-ups on a long credenza or bureau. If your counter is short add a roll-up under your torso.

- Lean over the counter from the hip crease, and place your head and crossed arms on the roll-up.

- Rest here as long as you like, with your head facing the side. Or if you like, add another blanket or towel to the roll-up so you can rest your forehead on it and still be able to breathe. The face-down option is easier on a tight neck.

- You may have to experiment with the height of the roll-up, but the effort is more than worth it. This pose is terrific for an aching upper or lower back!

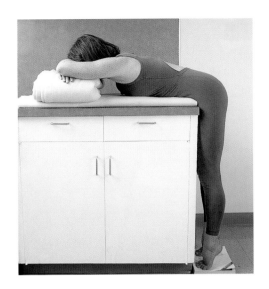

Hanging off the Couch

- Climb onto the couch and from your hip crease lean over the arm of the couch.

- Just hang there as long as you like, relaxing completely and allowing the tension to melt away.

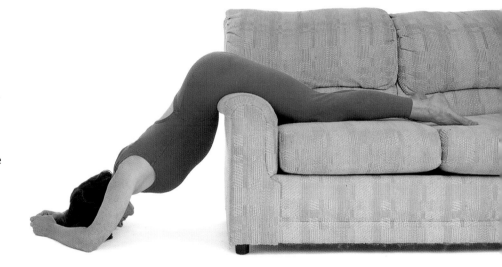

Chair Corpse Pose

- Lie on the floor with your calves on the chair seat.

- Place a blanket under your head if you like.

- Cover your eyes with a small towel or with your yoga tie and insert earplugs if you wish.

- With each exhalation, relax a little bit more.

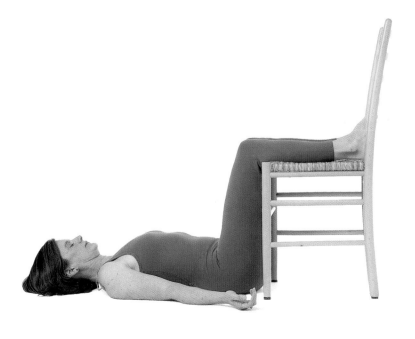

Rx for the Weekend Warrior

Certainly I am not the only one who spends my weekend overdoing. Whether it is skiing, hiking, playing tennis, gardening, or simply doing the weekend chores — we all try to get as much in on the weekend as possible. Monday morning rolls around and instead of feeling rejuvenated and ready to go back to work, we crave a massage or a hot tub.

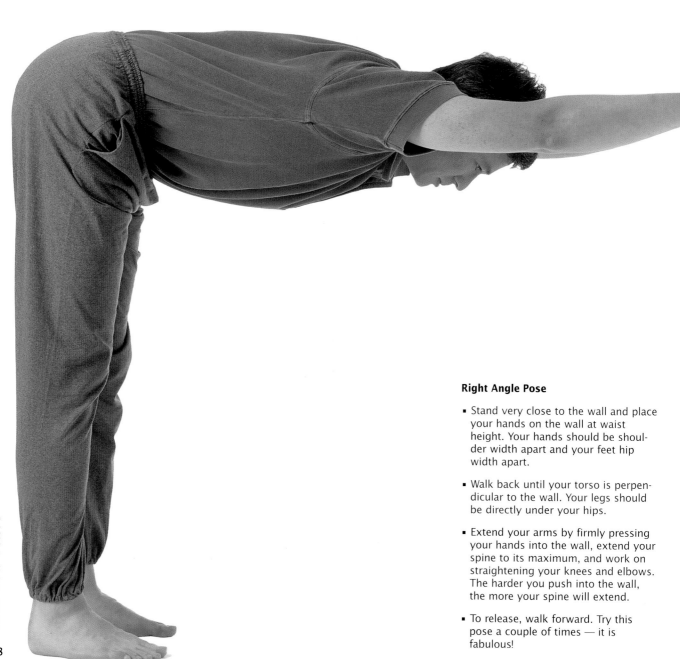

Right Angle Pose

- Stand very close to the wall and place your hands on the wall at waist height. Your hands should be shoulder width apart and your feet hip width apart.

- Walk back until your torso is perpendicular to the wall. Your legs should be directly under your hips.

- Extend your arms by firmly pressing your hands into the wall, extend your spine to its maximum, and work on straightening your knees and elbows. The harder you push into the wall, the more your spine will extend.

- To release, walk forward. Try this pose a couple of times — it is fabulous!

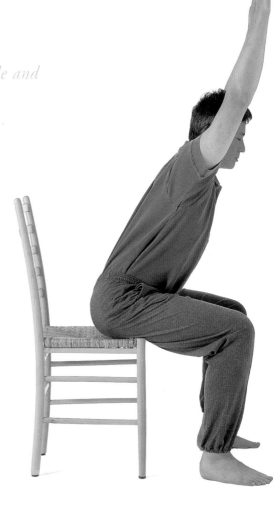

Upward Arm Stretch

- Sit in the chair facing the wall.

- Place your hands as high on the wall as possible and walk your fingers higher up the wall, stretching as though you are stretching from the lower back.

- Broaden your shoulders by separating and lifting your shoulder blades. Keep your neck and throat soft and don't tense your shoulders, just lift them.

- Once you think your fingers are as high as they can be, walk them a little higher.

Forward Arm Stretch

- Lie down on your stomach, facing the back of the chair.

- Place your hands as high on the chair as possible — the top, the sides, or the seat.

- Broaden your shoulders by separating your shoulder blades; work on straightening your elbows.

- If this is too easy or your elbows are not straight, scoot your body away from the chair.

- Lift the front legs of the chair, scoot the chair forward a little, and then try to push the front legs down to the floor.

Legs-up-the-Wall
Staff and Wide Angle Poses

- Lie down with your buttocks at the wall (or at least as close as possible).

- Extend your legs up the wall. Flex your toes toward you and work on getting your knees straight by extending the hamstrings.

- After a minute or so, widen your legs. Go slowly — you don't want to overstretch your inner thigh muscles!

- Flex your feet toward you.

- You can place rolled up blankets under your upper thighs to help support your legs. You will be able to stay in the pose longer this way.

- Keep flexing your feet toward you and trying to straighten your knees.

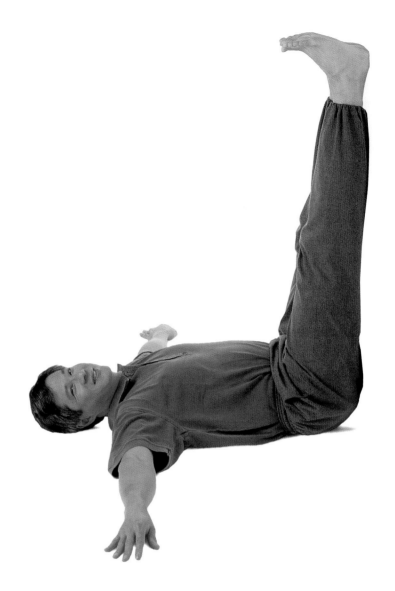

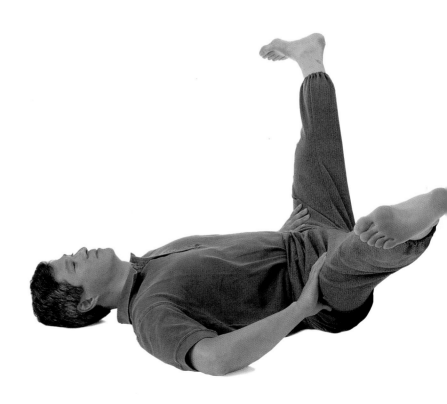

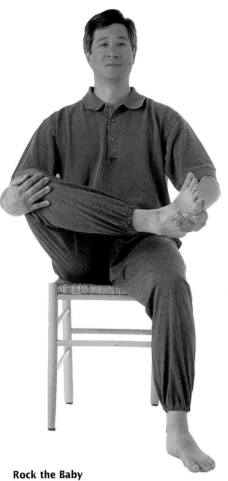

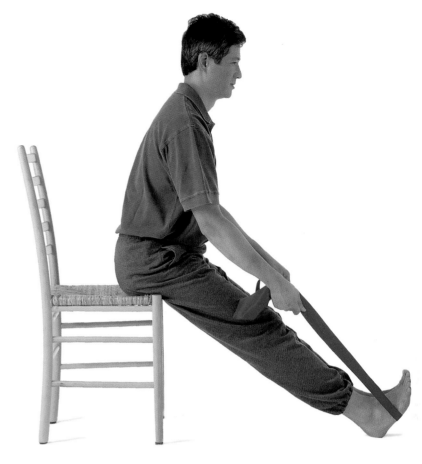

Rock the Baby

- Sit in the middle of the chair seat, keeping your back as straight as possible.

- Bring your right leg up, close to your chest.

- Place your knee in your right hand and your foot in your left hand.

- Bring your calf as close to your chest and as parallel to the floor as possible.

- Move your leg from side to side, as though you are rocking a baby.

- If you want a little more challenge, place your knee in the crook of one elbow, and your foot in the crook of the other elbow.

Chair Lower Back Stretch

- Sit in your chair and widen your legs so they are wider than hip distance apart.

- From the hip crease, bend forward and allow your entire body to relax. Drop your head and completely relax your neck.

- If you are not completely comfortable, try putting a rolled blanket or towel at your hip crease and lean over again.

Seated Double Hamstring Stretch

- Sit near the edge of the chair and place your feet on the wall, keeping your knees straight.

- Lengthen your back and lift your sternum. From the hip crease, lean forward.

- Only go as far forward as you can with your back straight.

- Hold onto the sides of the chair or use a tie around the balls of your feet for leverage.

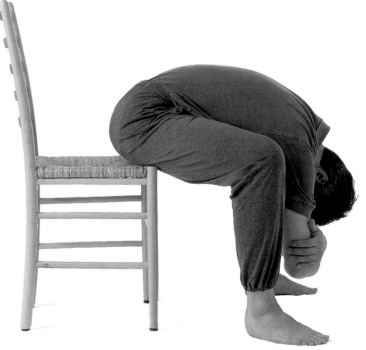

Oh, My Aching Feet!

The poor feet! We stand on them, we walk on them — all day, every day — carrying all of our weight. Sometimes we even make them run. And even though we may stretch our leg muscles to make running easier for them, we forget about stretching our feet, which are doing most of the work. Many of us even expect our feet to conform to shoes that make us look good, without caring how our feet feel about such abuse. And then, as if out of the blue, our feet will protest and start aching with a vengeance.

If you find yourself in such a predicament, try these foot exercises and soon you will find that your feet worship the ground you walk on.

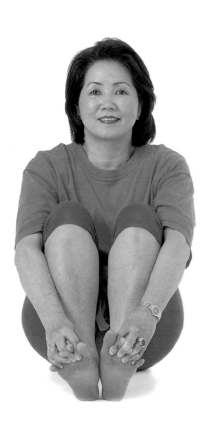

Fingers Between Toes

- Intertwine your fingers between your toes.

- Flex your feet toward you and squeeze your hand around your foot.

- You can do one foot at a time or both at once.

Foot in Arch Stretch

- Kneel with your knees and feet together.

- Place the top of your right foot into the arch of your left foot.

- Sit back on your feet.

- Once you've endured enough, switch feet.

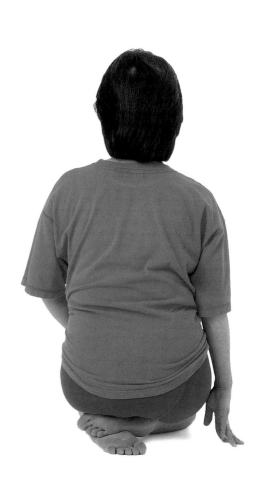

Feet Sitting

- Kneel with your legs, feet, and ankles together.

- Curl your toes under — making sure you get the little ones, too — and sit back on your heels.

- To decrease the intensity, keep your fingers on the floor.

- To intensify the stretch, tie a necktie around your ankles to hold them together.

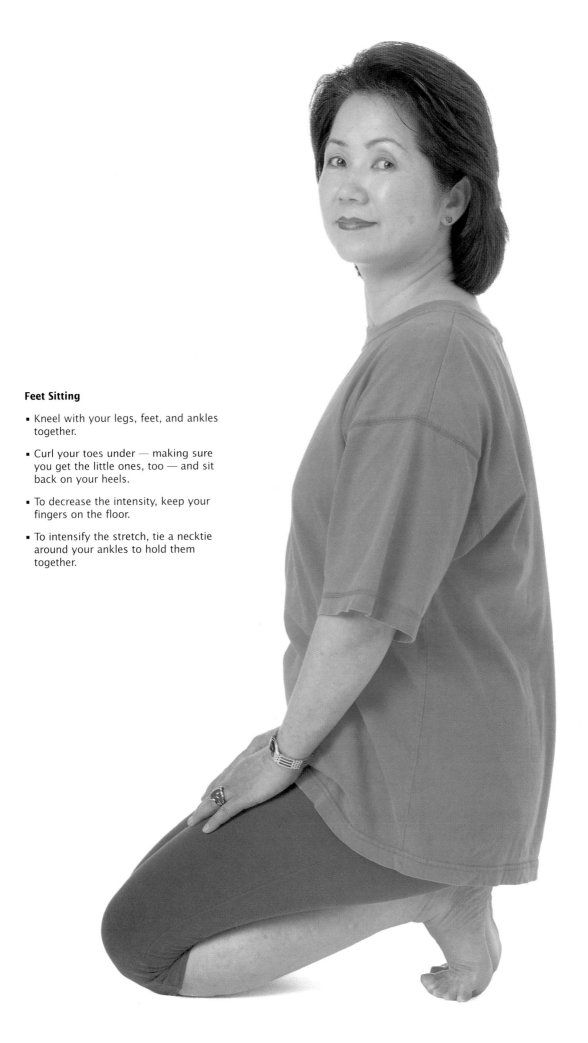

Calf Stretch 1

- Face the wall and place your hands on the wall at shoulder height.

- Position the toes and the ball of your left foot on the wall. Move your right foot back 2 to 3 feet.

- Slowly bend your left knee until you feel the stretch in your right calf.

- Lean into the wall to intensify the stretch.

- Switch sides.

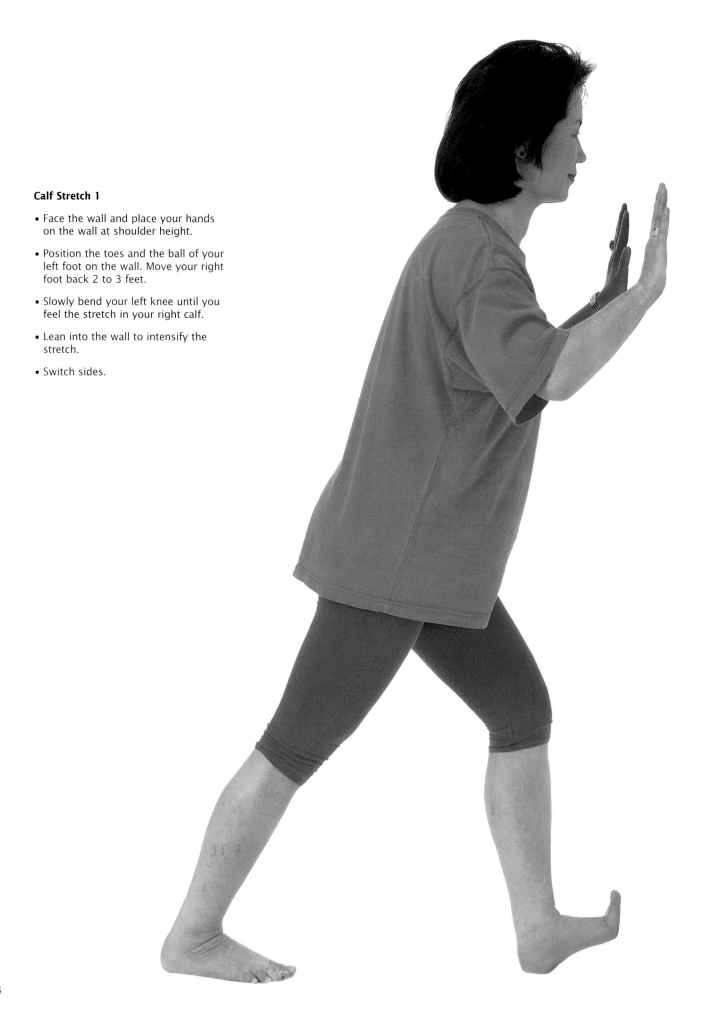

Calf Stretch 2

- Place a very thick book at the wall.

- Place the ball of your left foot on the book and move your right foot back just a few inches.

- Lean into the wall and allow the heel of your left foot to come down toward the floor.

- After a few moments, switch feet or do both feet at once.

- You can also do this pose on a step.

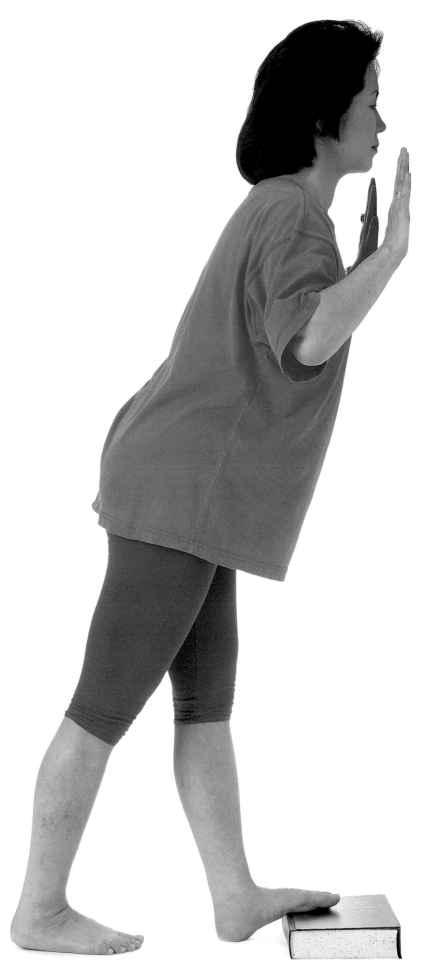

Slaying the Stress Monster

How often do we find ourselves having to maintain a calm exterior but ready to explode with stress on the inside? Frequently this happens at work and we have no immediate outlet for the stress. So what do we do? Maybe we have another cup of coffee or a cigarette, thinking this will help. We soon find that we were **wrong** and now we've increased our stress tenfold, so we take a couple of aspirin. This helps a little, but then what? Unfortunately, most of us have to wait until we get home to release some of this stress. So next time, instead of your favorite cocktail in front of the nightly news, try this routine and slay that stress monster, don't feed it!

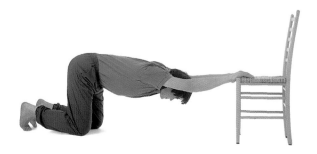

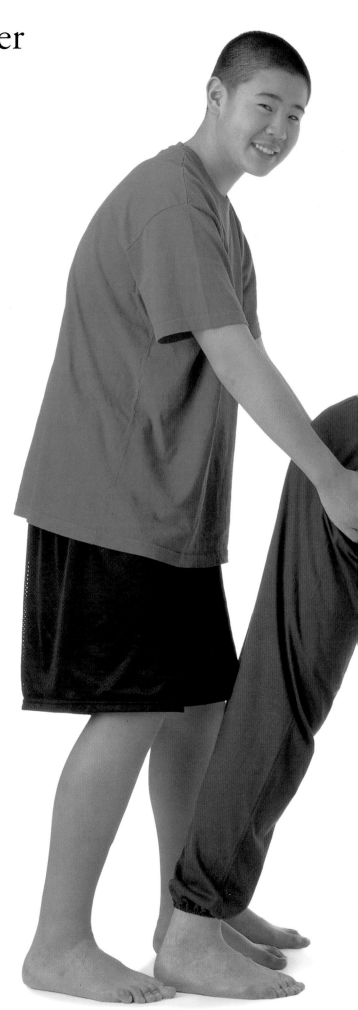

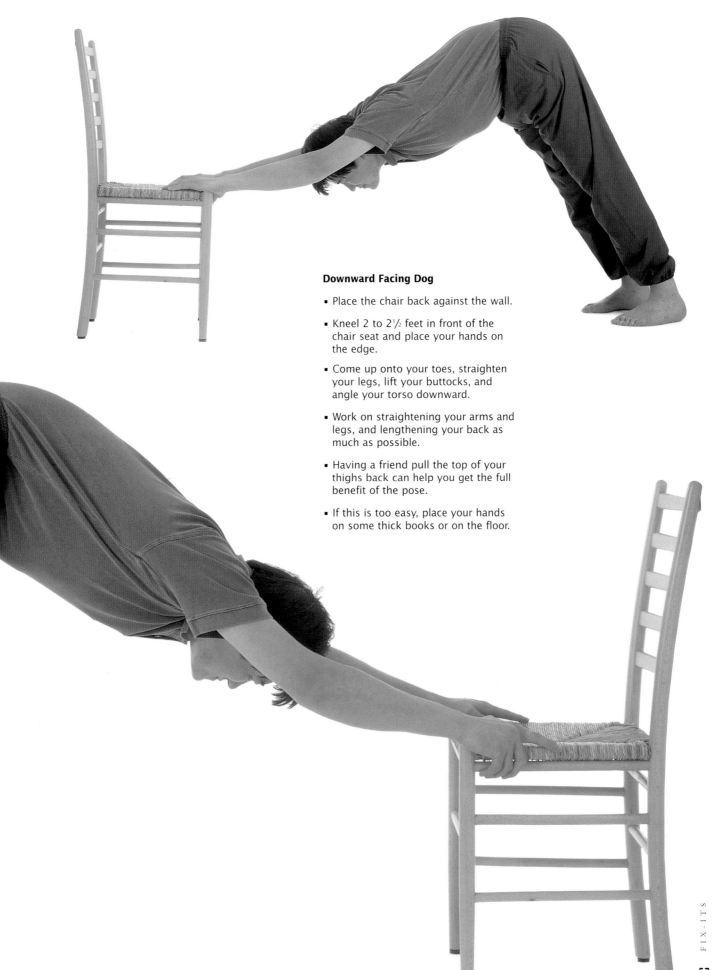

Downward Facing Dog

- Place the chair back against the wall.

- Kneel 2 to 2½ feet in front of the chair seat and place your hands on the edge.

- Come up onto your toes, straighten your legs, lift your buttocks, and angle your torso downward.

- Work on straightening your arms and legs, and lengthening your back as much as possible.

- Having a friend pull the top of your thighs back can help you get the full benefit of the pose.

- If this is too easy, place your hands on some thick books or on the floor.

Pre-Elbow Balance

- Place a dictionary against the wall, with the spine of the book facing you.

- Kneel down, placing your thumbs in front of the book and your index fingers on the side of it. Your forearms are on the floor and your elbows are directly under your shoulders.

- Then, come up on your toes, straightening your knees if you can, and walk in toward the wall.

- Keep lifting your shoulders—to your absolute maximum—and walk in a little more.

- Allow your head to hang down toward the floor.

- You can have a friend stand at the wall, bend his or her knees, and place them in your back, just below your shoulder blades. This will help you lift your shoulders, giving you the sense of how the pose will feel when you are lifting your shoulders to your maximum.

- Hold the pose as long as you can. Initially this may only be a few seconds.

- Rest for a few moments and try again.

- Another trick is to tie a necktie around your arms, an inch above your elbows, to help keep your arms in place and make the pose a little easier.

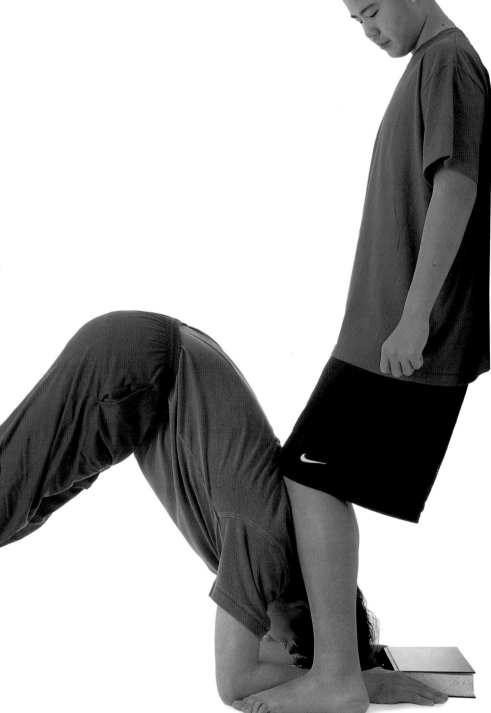

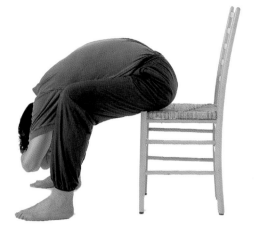

Chair Lower Back Stretch

- Sit in your chair and widen your legs so they are wider than hip distance apart.

- From the hip crease, bend forward and allow your entire body to relax. Drop your head and completely relax your neck.

- If you are not completely comfortable, try putting a rolled blanket or towel at the hip crease and lean over again.

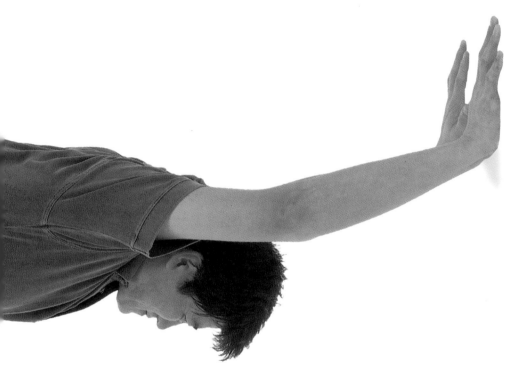

Warrior III

- Return to Right Angle Pose — placing your hands on the wall at waist height and walking your feet back until your legs and torso form a right angle. Push into the wall to extend your arms and spine.

- Shift your weight to your left leg.

- Now—extend your right leg straight behind you, keeping your leg even with your hips and your front hipbones even, and flex your toes toward you. Perhaps you need an assistant!

- Bring your leg down, re-establish Right Angle Pose, and then extend your left leg.

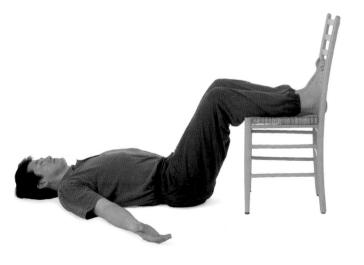

Chair Corpse Pose

- Lie on the floor with your calves on the chair seat.

- Place a pillow or blanket under your head if you like.

- Cover your eyes with a small towel or with your yoga tie and insert earplugs if you wish.

- With each exhalation, relax a little bit more.

I'm Fried!

Everyone knows this feeling. We are absolutely beat. Zero energy. All we want to do is crawl into bed and sleep for a week. But because this is not a possibility, try the following poses as an alternative. You may fall asleep in the Passive Backbend Series. Whether you sleep or not, you will soon feel completely refreshed.

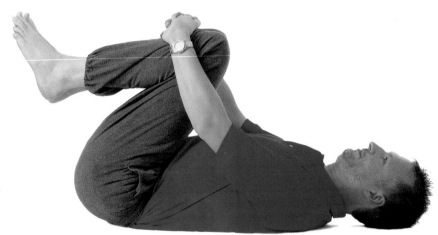

Knees to Chest

- Lie on your back, bring your knees into your chest, and hug them.

- Breathe deeply into your lower back and with each exhalation, allow your entire back to relax just a little bit more.

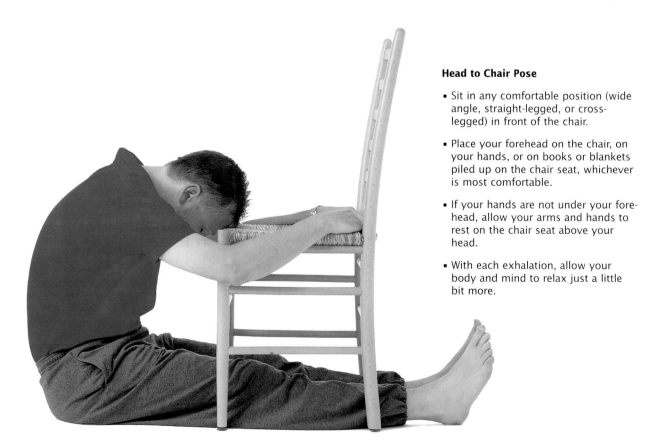

Head to Chair Pose

- Sit in any comfortable position (wide angle, straight-legged, or cross-legged) in front of the chair.

- Place your forehead on the chair, on your hands, or on books or blankets piled up on the chair seat, whichever is most comfortable.

- If your hands are not under your forehead, allow your arms and hands to rest on the chair seat above your head.

- With each exhalation, allow your body and mind to relax just a little bit more.

Passive Backbend Series

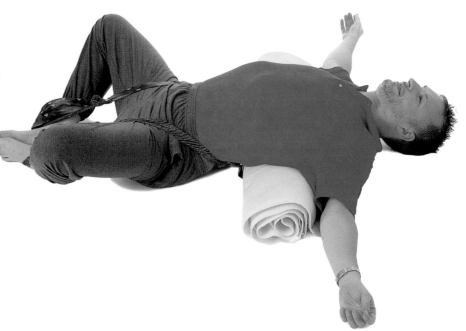

- Roll up a blanket or two and place the roll right behind your sternum. Determine if you like the height or not, then adjust accordingly. You can also try placing folded blankets under your head, neck, and shoulders to determine if that is more comfortable.

- Sitting in front of your blanket setup, take two neckties that are knotted together on one end. Come into Bound Angle Pose:

  - Bring the soles of your feet together.

  - Place the tie around your lower back, over the top of your right thigh and calf, around the outside of your feet, and on top of your left thigh and calf. Knot the necktie with the knot falling between your calf and thigh. The tie should be taut but not so tight that you will have no mobility when you lie down.

  - Then lie back over your blanket roll so the roll supports your middle back. If your lower back hurts, place a thick book under your feet.

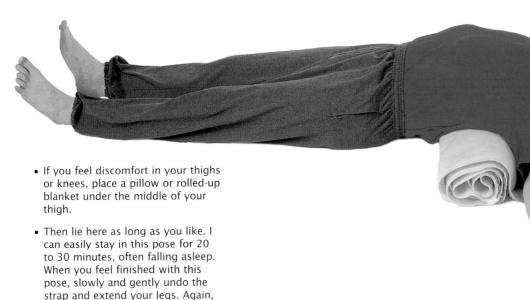

- If you feel discomfort in your thighs or knees, place a pillow or rolled-up blanket under the middle of your thigh.

- Then lie here as long as you like. I can easily stay in this pose for 20 to 30 minutes, often falling asleep. When you feel finished with this pose, slowly and gently undo the strap and extend your legs. Again, stay in this pose as long as you like.

- When you are ready, roll over to your right or left side, and stay there until you are ready to roll over to the other side. You may need an extra blanket on hand for your head. Or you can use your arm as an extra lift.

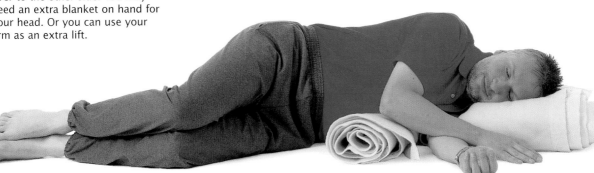

Boy, What a Pain in the Neck!

There is often something that gives us a pain in the neck, like our 16-year-old wrecking the car, or unwelcome projects at work. If you have a neckache or a headache, try this series of poses and see how quickly relief will come.

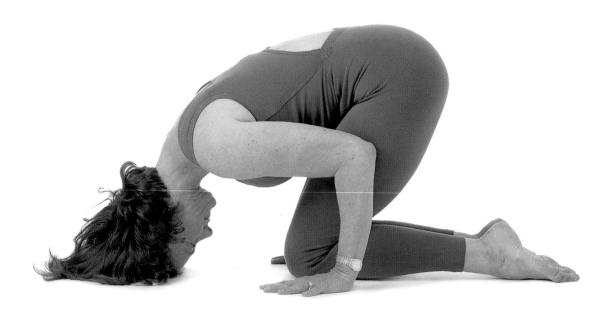

Head Roll

This should be done on a carpeted floor, or use a thick towel or blanket.

- Kneel on all fours and place your head on the floor.

- Then slowly roll your head forward toward your forehead and then backward toward the crown of your head.

- This will activate the pressure points on the top of your head and help ease the pain in your head and neck.

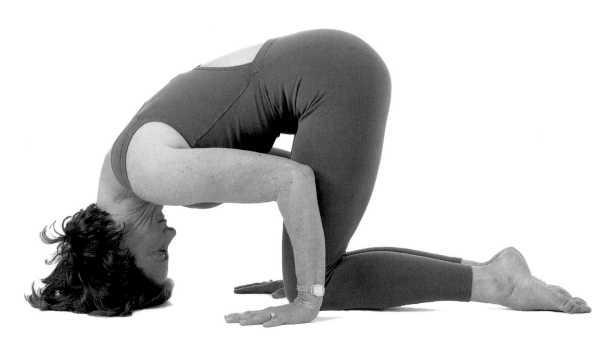

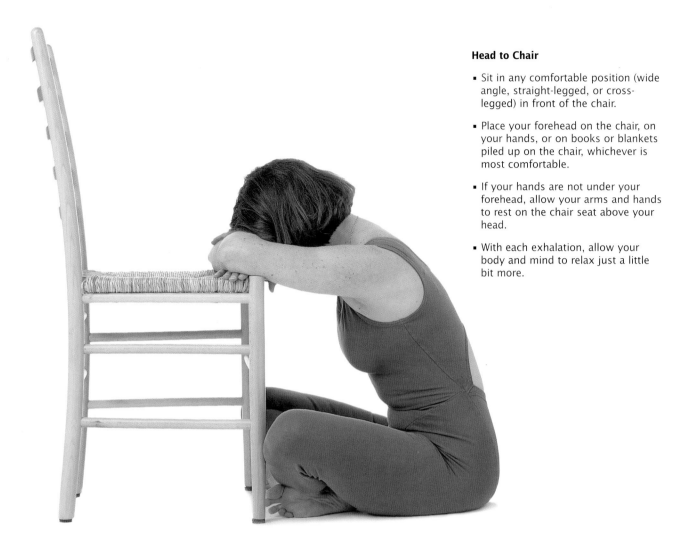

Head to Chair

- Sit in any comfortable position (wide angle, straight-legged, or cross-legged) in front of the chair.

- Place your forehead on the chair, on your hands, or on books or blankets piled up on the chair, whichever is most comfortable.

- If your hands are not under your forehead, allow your arms and hands to rest on the chair seat above your head.

- With each exhalation, allow your body and mind to relax just a little bit more.

Book Support

- Place a dictionary or other thick book on the floor.

- Lie on your back, placing your head on the book. Your knees are bent and together and your feet are wider than hip distance. If you are not completely comfortable, experiment with the thickness or the placement of the book.

- You will be surprised how quickly relaxation comes in this pose.

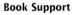

Alternatives for the Couch Potato, or Poses to Do While Watching TV

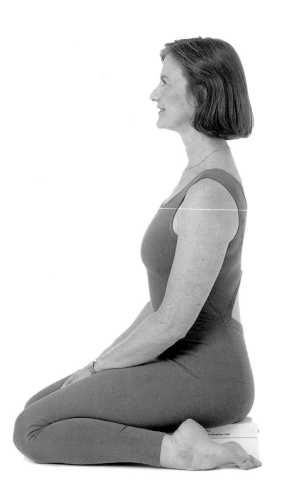

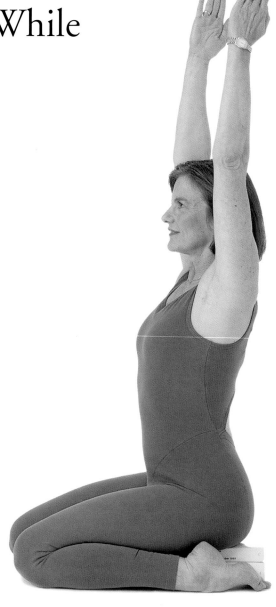

Hero Series

- Place a thick book on the floor.

- Kneel, with your knees hip distance apart, in front of the book.

- Roll your calves outward and sit on the book.

- If you are immediately uncomfortable, come up and add another book.

- If your ankles are unhappy, roll up some small face towels and place them under your ankles. You may have to experiment with the thickness of the rolls.

Arm Variations 1

- Stretch your arms straight overhead, palms facing each other.

- Lengthen your arms as though you are stretching all the way from the hips.

- Lift your sternum and keep reaching for the ceiling.

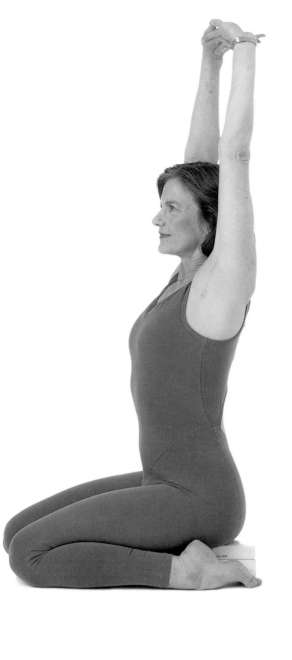

Finally, something constructive to do while watching our favorite TV programs. No more guilt about being a couch potato. We are gaining flexibility and accomplishing our yoga goals — not wasting our time!

Arm Variations 2

- Interlock your fingers, turn your palms outward, and stretch your arms overhead.

- Keep your thumbs even with your hands and work on straightening your elbows.

- Release, change the interlock (in other words, interlock your fingers the uncomfortable way) and extend your arms again.

Arm Variations 3

- Bring your arms behind your back, holding a tie between your hands.

- Lift your arms only as high as you can. Keep your sternum lifted and your arms straight.

- As you gain flexibility, move your hands closer on the tie. Or dispense with the tie and interlock your fingers.

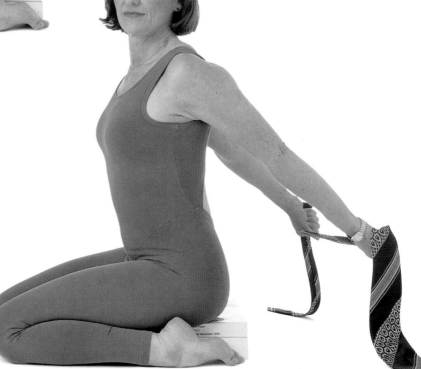

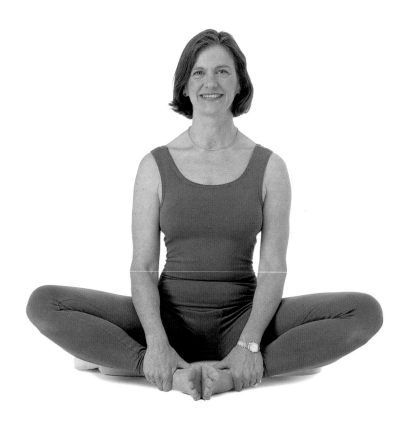

Bound Angle Pose

- Sit on the floor or on folded blankets next to the wall or couch.

- Extend your legs in front of you, bend your right knee, and bring your foot to the center of your body.

- Then bend your left knee, in the same fashion, and bring your left foot to meet the right foot, placing the soles of your feet together.

- If your knees are higher than your waist, add more blankets until your knees are at or below your waist.

- Lengthen your spine and lift your sternum.

  To help straighten your spine, place your hands or fingertips on the floor beside you (if you are sitting on a prop, you may have to place your hands on books that are placed behind you) and lift your torso.

- As always, remember to keep your throat, neck, and shoulders relaxed as you lift your spine.

- Firmly press the soles of your feet together. This will automatically help extend your inner thighs and outer thighs toward the knees and open your inner hip joints.

- The objective of this pose is not to get your knees to the floor, but rather to extend your thighs so you can gain flexibility in the inner and the outer thighs, and the hips.

Seated Wide Angle Pose

- Sit on some folded blankets or against the couch.

- Stretch your legs out to the side.

- Lengthen your back and lift your sternum.

- Keeping your back straight, bend slightly forward from the hip crease.

Important Note: *Bend forward only to the degree you can keep your back straight. For most of us this is not very far!*

Cow Pose

- Kneel on all fours with your hands directly under your shoulders and your knees directly under your hips.

- Cross your left knee behind your right knee

- Keeping your knees close together, move your feet out to each side.

- Slowly sit on the floor. If you can't reach the floor, sit on a book or blanket.

- If the right knee comes up high, place a book under your foot.

- When you are ready, come out of the pose onto all fours again, and switch the cross of your knees.

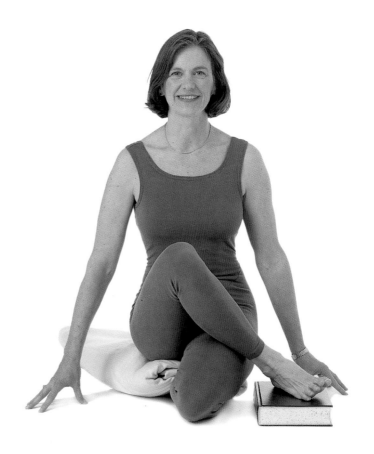

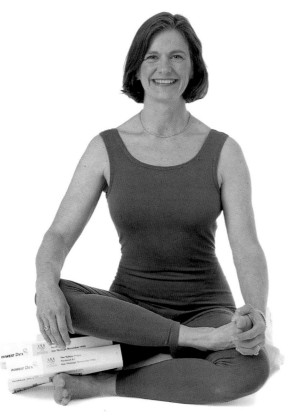

Pre-Lotus

- Sit with your back at the wall or a couch and your legs extended.

- Bend your left knee and place your calf so it is parallel to the wall or couch.

- Bend your right knee and place your right foot on your left knee. Extend your lower back and lift your sternum.

- If your right knee is far from your left foot, place a book or blanket between your foot and knee.

- Hold as long as you like and switch sides.

Down in the Dumps

*Let's face it. From time to time
we all get "down in the dumps."
We get sick, we lose our jobs,
our relationships go south, our
loved ones die, or we are trying
to heal the emotional traumas
of the past. Presented here is a
series of poses that will help
heal your emotions as well as
your body. Try this routine next
time you simply want to hide
and cry.*

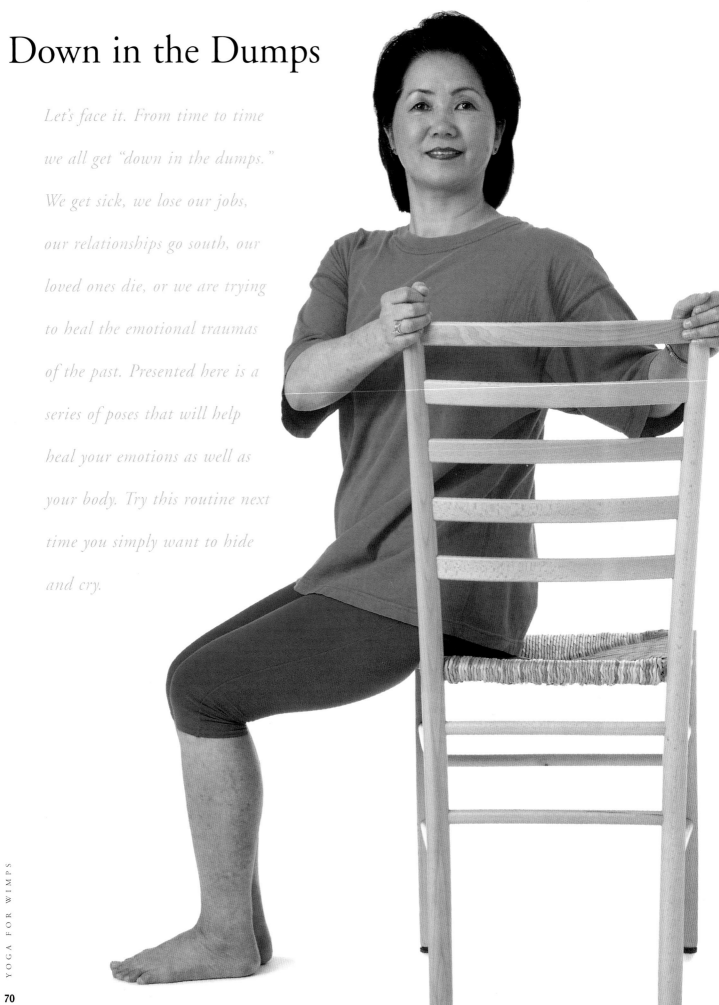

Chair Twist 1 (left page)

- Sit on the *edge* of your chair sideways with your left side facing the chair back.

- Firmly plant your feet on the floor. Make sure your feet and knees remain together and even throughout the pose.

- Place your hands on the chair as shown.

- On an inhalation straighten your spine and on an exhalation twist toward the chair, twisting from the very bottom of your spine — pushing with your right hand and pulling with your left hand.

- Repeat the inhalation/straighten, exhalation/twist series several times.

- Release and switch sides.

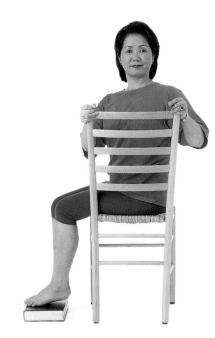

Chair Twist 2

- Sit in the *middle* of your chair sideways with your left side facing the chair back.

- Repeat the same routine as in Chair Twist 1.

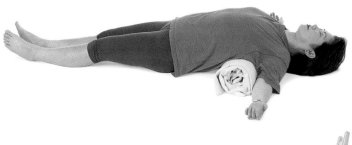

Supported Chest Opener

- Roll up a blanket or thick towel. Lie down with the roll placed under your upper middle back.

- If you would like, use a pillow or folded blanket under your head.

- Close your eyes and relax.

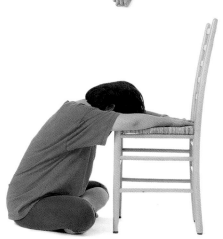

Head to Chair

- Sit in any comfortable position (wide angle, straight-legged, or cross-legged) in front of the chair.

- Place your forehead on the chair, on your hands, or on books or blankets piled up on the chair, whichever is most comfortable.

- With each exhalation, allow your body and mind to relax just a little bit more.

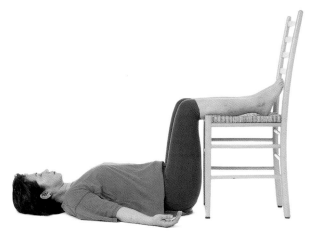

Chair Corpse Pose

- Lie on the floor with your calves on the chair seat.

- Place a pillow or blanket under your head if you like.

- Cover your eyes with a small towel or with your yoga tie and insert earplugs if you wish.

- With each exhalation, relax a little bit more.

As you progress and want more information and

challenge, check out this section. It gives detailed

instructions, suggests time periods for holding

each pose, and is organized so you can practice

each group of poses as a series.

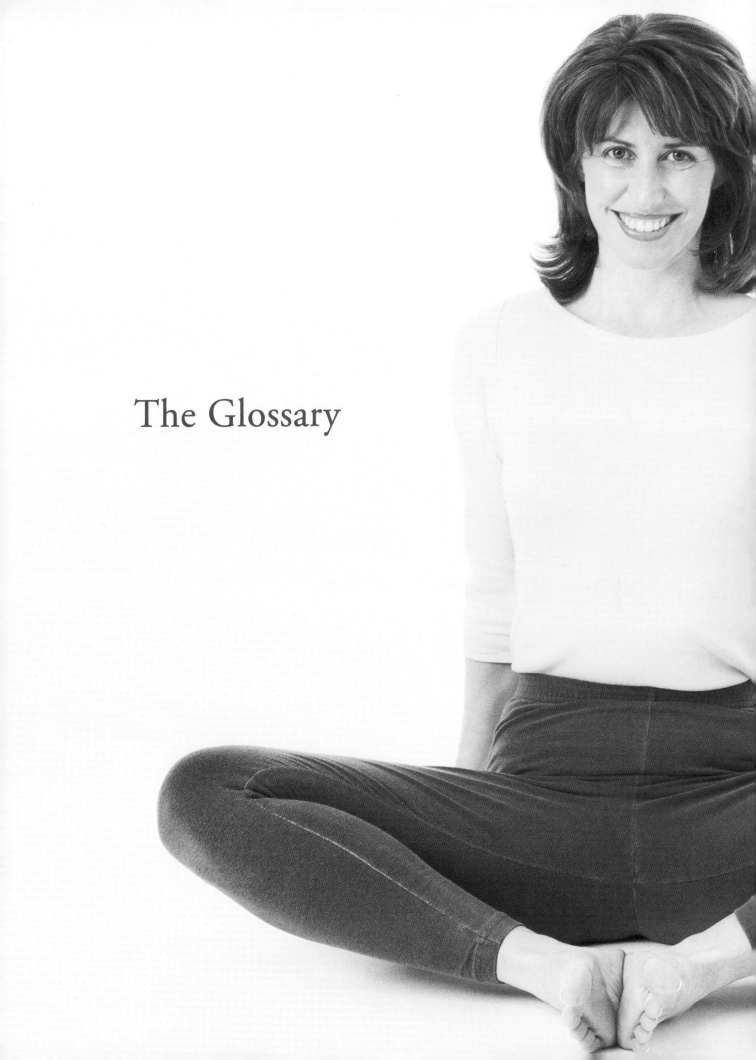

The Glossary

Legs-up-the-Wall Poses

This series of poses is good to do if you are tired and don't want to exert yourself or if your back aches a little and you just want pampering. You may also find, though, that if you do these poses, you will have the energy to do another series that requires a little more effort.

The following poses are traditionally done sitting on the floor. In this series, however, we lie on the floor and use the wall as a prop. This method makes the poses much easier to do: gravity is your friend! So, if you have tight hamstrings (the muscles on the backs of your thighs) and inner thigh muscles, try these poses before you try the traditional poses, and use the suggested props.

These poses will increase flexibility in the hamstrings, inner thighs, and hips and help relieve back, knee, and ankle problems.

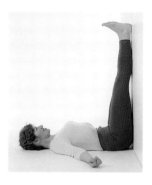

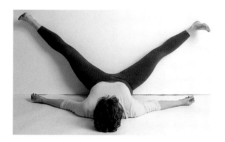

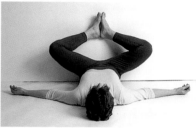

STAFF POSE

Lie on your back with your buttocks at the wall (or as close to the wall as possible) and your legs up the wall. Your knees are straight — or at least you are trying to straighten them! Press your legs toward the wall. You can place your hands on the top of your thighs to help you press your legs into the wall until you get the feel of this on your own. Your feet should be perfectly parallel with the ceiling, so flex your toes toward your face.

Cautions/Hints
If you can't straighten your knees or if you can't align yourself directly against the wall, place an old necktie around the balls of your feet, holding one end of the tie in each hand. With your toes flexed toward your face, press your feet into the tie — this provides resistance. Keep practicing — the hamstrings will loosen!

WIDE ANGLE POSE

Starting from Staff Pose, with your legs straight up the wall, allow your legs to move down the wall away from each other so they form a "V." Continue to press your thighs against the wall, using your hands to press them if necessary. Your knees are straight or as close to straight as possible. Flex your toes toward your face. Allow gravity to help you form a more obtuse angle.

Stay as long as you like, increasing the time as you progress.

Cautions/Hints
Go slowly! You do not want to overstretch your inner thigh muscles. If you are very stiff, support your outer thighs with your hands or place rolled-up blankets under the top of each thigh. The blanket setup will help release your inner thighs slowly as the muscles soften.

BOUND ANGLE POSE

From Wide Angle Pose, bring the soles of your feet together and press them together firmly. Do not use your hands to press your knees toward the wall! Lengthen your tailbone toward the wall (at least, imagine it is moving toward the wall until you can actually feel that it is moving). Stay in this pose as long as possible, using the force of gravity to help you ease into it.

Cautions/Hints
I repeat, do not use your hands to press your knees toward the wall!

Seated Poses

These poses increase flexibility in the hips, thighs, and lower back and help you build lower back strength. Some of the poses include arm stretches, which increase flexibility in the arms, shoulders, and upper back — doubling the benefits.

In this series, sitting on a folded blanket or two is often suggested. This gives support to the lower back and helps reduce stiffness in the thighs. If you are uncomfortable on the floor, try sitting on the folded blankets. You will be glad you did!

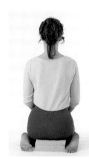

HERO SERIES

Kneel on the floor with a thick book behind you. Lean forward, and use your hands to roll your calves outward. Then sit back on the prop, releasing your hands at the last possible second before sitting. Now that you are seated, bring your knees together. Sit up as straight as possible. Lengthen your lower back and lift your sternum. Soften your throat, neck, and shoulders.

Cautions/Hints

If your knees or ankles hurt, add another book. If your ankles are uncomfortable, but your knees are okay, place rolled-up face cloths under them. Experiment with the thickness of the roll and determine if you need support for one ankle or two. If you have had a history of knee problems, place the rolled-up face cloth behind the sensitive knee. Again, experiment with thickness.

This is a terrific exercise for invigorating the legs. It helps to heal knee problems, improve circulation, reduce varicose veins, and improve low arches or flat feet. For these benefits, you must hold the pose for at least 10 minutes a day. To keep boredom at bay, try some of these arm exercises.

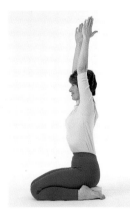

ARM VARIATION 1

Raise your arms overhead, palms facing each other. Stretch your arms as though you are stretching all the way from your waist, keeping your throat, neck, and shoulders relaxed.

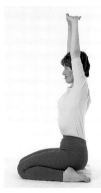

ARM VARIATION 2

Interlock your hands and turn your palms outward. Extend your arms in front of you, elbows straight, and stretch all the way from the shoulders. Slowly bring your arms over your head. Again, stretch from your waist and keep your throat, neck, and shoulders relaxed.

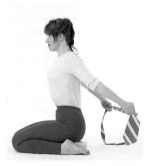

ARM VARIATION 3

Bring your hands behind your back and hold a tie between them. Allow your hands to separate to a point that is comfortable for your shoulders, but not so comfortable that you don't feel a stretch. As you gain flexibility, you will be able to tighten up on the tie and bring your hands higher, and eventually dispense with the tie!

SEATED BOUND ANGLE POSE

Sit on the floor next to a wall or on a folded blanket with your legs straight in front of you. Placing your right hand under your right knee, bend your right knee and bring your foot to the center of your body. Then bend your left knee, in the same fashion, and bring your left foot to meet your right foot, placing the soles of your feet together. Lengthen your spine and lift your sternum. Relax your throat, neck, and shoulders. To help straighten your spine, place your hands or fingertips on the floor beside you (if you are sitting on a prop, you may have to place your hands on books that are placed behind you) and lift your torso. Firmly press the soles of your feet together—this will automatically help extend your inner and outer thighs toward your knees and open your hip joints.

*The objective of this pose is **not** to get your knees to the floor,* but rather to extend your thighs so you can gain flexibility in the inner thighs, the outer thighs, and the hips. The more you press the soles of your feet together, the more naturally this action will occur.

Hold as long as you can, increasing the time as you progress.

Cautions/Hints
If your knees are above your waist, add folded blankets until your knees are even with or below your waist. If this pose seems too difficult, try it with your legs up the wall, as described on page 75. This pose gives energy, increases flexibility in the thighs and hips, and helps relieve kidney or urinary tract problems. Pregnant women should sit in this pose several minutes a day to help ease pain during delivery.

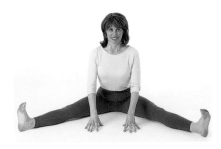

SEATED WIDE ANGLE POSE

Sit on the floor or on some folded blankets with your legs fully extended. Stretch your legs outward so they are in a "V." Straighten your knees as much as possible by extending your hamstrings. Make sure your feet are flexed toward you. Lengthen your lower back and lift your sternum. Soften your throat, neck, and shoulders. Lengthen your spine by placing your fingertips on the floor — either beside you or behind you — and press them into the floor. Check your posture again and adjust or relax where necessary.

Place your hands a few inches in front of you, and from the hip crease, slowly bend forward, walking your hands forward as far as you can. Breathe as you bend forward. Make sure your back is straight and extended. Lifting the sternum will help straighten your upper back.

Cautions/Hints
If this pose is too difficult, try the Legs-Up-the-Wall version on page 75.

ANGLE VARIATION (below)

Start from Seated Wide Angle Pose. Lengthen your lower back and lift your sternum. Slightly twist your torso toward your right leg, and place this around the ball of your foot. Try to align the center of your chest with your right leg. (This may be impossible to do, but use this alignment as a goal.) From the hip crease slightly bend over the right leg. Only bend as far forward as you can with your back straight. Continue to adjust your posture — lengthening your back and lifting your sternum.

Once you've gone as far as you can, hold for 30 to 45 seconds, increasing the time as you progress. Release and switch sides.

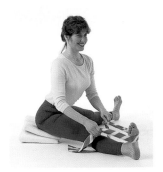

PRE-LOTUS

Sit with your back at the wall or at the couch and your legs extended. Bend your left knee and place your calf so it is parallel to the wall or couch. Bend your right knee and place your right foot on your left knee. Flex both feet. Extend your lower back and lift your sternum. If your left knee is far from your right foot, place a book or blanket between your foot and knee. Hold as long as you like and switch sides.

Cautions/Hints
If your hips are stiff, sit on a folded blanket.

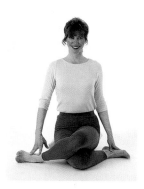

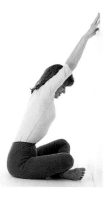

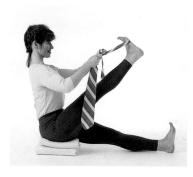

COW POSE

Kneel on all fours with your hands directly under your shoulders and your knees directly under your hips. Cross your right knee behind your left knee. Keeping your knees close together, move your feet out to your sides. Slowly sit on the floor. If you can't reach the floor, place a book or blanket under your buttocks. If your right knee comes up high, place a book under your foot. When you are ready, come out of the pose onto all fours again, and switch the cross of your knees.

Cautions/Hints

If you feel sharp knee pain, increase the height of the props. If that doesn't stop the pain, sit on one of your legs and add a blanket or book under the other leg. (Hip pain is okay here!) Sitting in this pose allows your back to lift and straighten naturally, giving a tremendous sense of strength, power, and well-being.

CROSS-LEGGED LOWER BACK STRETCH

Sit a few inches from the wall, facing it, with your legs crossed. Place your hands as high on the wall as you can. Broaden your shoulders by separating your shoulder blades. Walk your fingers up the wall, stretching from the lower back. When you think you have gone as high as you can, rest for a moment while your body adjusts to the pose, and then walk your fingers a little higher. Rest and repeat several times.

Cautions/Hints

If this pose is too difficult, try Upward Arm Stretch on page 92 instead.

ARCHER POSE

Sit on the floor or on folded blankets with your legs extended straight in front of you and your feet at the wall. Bend your right knee and bring your leg in toward you. Place the tie around the ball of your right foot and, with your knee bent, place the sole of the foot on the floor. Lengthen your lower back and lift your sternum. Soften your throat, neck, and shoulders. Lift your right leg, straightening the knee if possible. Flex the raised foot toward you and press the foot of the extended leg into the wall. Lift your leg only to the point that you can keep it lifted with your back straight. Continue to adjust your posture in the pose, keeping your neck, throat, and shoulders soft.

Hold the pose for 30 to 45 seconds, increasing the time as you progress. Release and switch sides.

FULL FORWARD BEND

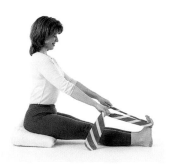

Sit on the floor or on some folded blankets, extend your legs in front of you, and flex your feet toward you. Strap the balls of your feet with a tie and hold one end of the tie in each hand, as close to your feet as possible without bending the spine. Move your thighs toward the floor, keeping your knees straight or working toward that by extending your hamstrings. Lengthen your lower back and lift your sternum. Relax your throat, neck, and shoulders. From the hip crease, slowly bend over your legs. Only bend as far forward as you can with your back straight. Keep lengthening your lower back muscles and lifting your sternum.

Hold the pose for 30 to 45 seconds, increasing the time as you progress.

Cautions/Hints

For people who have backs that curve outward, try to make the spine convex (bend inward). This will eventually help to bring the spine back to a normal curve.

Chair Forward Bends

We can work in forward bends or we can do them in a relaxing and restorative manner. This section contains both "working" and restorative forward bends. In addition to the obvious benefit of increased flexibility, when we "work" in forward bends we strengthen the lower back muscles. The correct action for working in forward bends is to lengthen your lower back and lift your sternum. As you bend from the hip crease, keep your back straight. Lifting your sternum upward helps straighten your upper back.

In many of the relaxing forward bends we allow our backs to round. These poses help quiet the mind and are beneficial to those suffering from either high or low blood pressure.

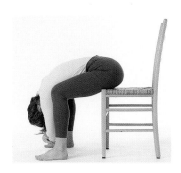

CHAIR LOWER BACK STRETCH

Sit near the edge of the chair seat, legs bent normally. Separate your legs so they are wider than hip distance apart. From the hip crease, bend forward. Drop your head completely and relax your neck and shoulders. Your back can round in this pose. Just hang in the pose, as though you are a rag doll. To further relax, hold your elbows. Allow your head to hang loosely, consciously releasing the tension in your neck. If you like, you can use the chair legs to pull your body forward and down.

Hold this pose as long as you like, allowing each exhalation to relax your body and your mind a little bit more. Sit up on an inhalation, pause for a few moments, and try again.

Cautions/Hints
I hear two complaints about this pose. The first is that the stomach gets in the way and the second is that the muscles at the top of the thighs tighten. For both problems, place a rolled-up towel or blanket at the very top of your thighs. Try to lift your stomach over it and lean forward again. This should eliminate any interference and the thighs should soften.

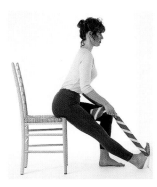

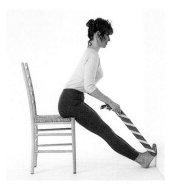

SEATED HAMSTRING STRETCH

Sit near the edge of the chair, facing the wall. Straighten your right leg and place your right heel on the floor and the ball of your right foot on the wall. Place a tie around the ball of your right foot. Your left leg is bent normally. Lengthen your lower back and lift your sternum. Soften your throat, neck, and shoulders. From the hip crease, lean forward toward the wall. Only bend as far forward as you can with your back straight.

Hold for 30 to 45 seconds, increasing the time as you progress. Release and switch sides.

Cautions/Hints
Lifting your sternum helps straighten your upper back.

SEATED DOUBLE HAMSTRING STRETCH

Sit near the edge of the chair and place both feet on the wall, legs straight. Place a tie around the ball of your feet. Lengthen your lower back and lift your sternum. Soften your throat, neck, and shoulders. From the hip crease, lean forward toward the wall. Only bend as far forward as you can with your back straight.

Cautions/Hints
Lifting your sternum helps straighten your upper back.

BENCH FORWARD BEND

Sit near the edge of the bench or chair, legs extended forward with both feet on the wall. From the hip crease, lean forward over your legs. Keep your knees straight, if you can. Place a blanket at the point on your legs where your forehead would fall if you were that flexible. At this point, you can bend your knees and round your back. Place your forehead on the prop and allow your body to melt into the pose. Stay in this position as long as you like. Or release the pose and go back into it several times.

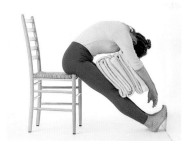

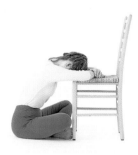

HEAD TO CHAIR POSE

Sit in any comfortable position in front of your chair. Place your forehead on the chair seat, on your hands, or on books or blankets stacked on the chair seat, whichever is most comfortable for you. If your forehead is not on your hands, place your arms and hands on the chair in front of your head. You can round your back in this pose. With each exhalation, allow your body and mind to relax just a little bit more. Stay in this pose as long as you like. When you are ready, slowly come up on an inhalation.

Cautions/Hints
The pressure on the forehead helps quiet the mind. This pose also helps relieve neck pain, headaches, and anxiety.

Lying-on-the-Floor Poses

These poses increase flexibility in the legs and help reduce stiffness in the lower back. You will recognize some of these poses from the Legs-up-the-Wall series, but without the wall the work is a little more intense. Don't worry; you will gain expertise (i.e., flexibility) as you practice.

Note: In the poses in which you hold a tie, be aware of how you are holding it — you don't have to hold on for dear life!

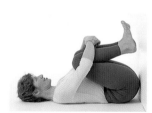

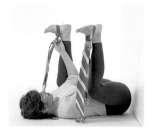

KNEES TO THE CHEST

Lying on the floor, bend your knees and bring them toward your chest, embracing your legs with your arms. Hug your legs. If you like, you can gently rock from side to side.

Cautions/Hints
If this is painful for your knees, roll up small face towels and place them behind your knees.

DEAD BUG POSE

Lie on your back and bend your legs so your knees are close to your armpits, your thighs are near the sides of your torso, and your calves are at right angles to your thighs. Your feet are positioned as if you will walk on the ceiling. Place a tie across the arch of each foot and pull your legs toward the floor. Try to keep your calves perpendicular to your thighs. Try to keep your tailbone moving toward the wall.

This pose feels terrific on a tight lower back and you can stay in it as long as you like!

Cautions/Hints
If this is easy, use your hands instead of the tie, clasping your arches from the inside of your thighs, and pulling your feet toward you.

RECLINING HAMSTRING STRETCH

Lie on your back with your feet at the wall, pressing them into the wall. Bring your right foot in toward your chest and strap the ball of this foot. Lift your leg and straighten your knee, flexing your toes toward you. Keep pressing your left foot into the wall. Try to straighten both knees by lengthening your hamstrings. A straight knee with a lower leg is better than a bent knee with a higher leg.

Hold for 30 to 45 seconds, increasing the time as you progress. Slowly release and switch sides.

Cautions/Hints
After doing both sides individually, place the tie around the balls of both feet, press your feet into the tie, and lift both legs. Try to straighten your knees, and keep your feet flexed toward you.

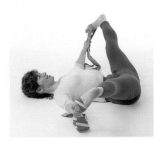

DOUBLE INNER THIGH STRETCH

Lie on your back with your legs extended and your feet flexed toward you. Bring both legs in toward your body and place a tie around the ball of each foot. Slowly allow your legs to release outward toward your shoulders. Try to keep both knees straight by extending your hamstrings. Keep both feet flexed toward you. If your inner thighs are very stiff, place a rolled-up blanket or very thick book under your upper thighs, thus allowing the inner thighs to relax more easily.

Hold for 20 to 30 seconds, increasing the time as you progress.

RECLINING INNER THIGH STRETCH

Lie on your back with your feet at the wall, pressing them into the wall. Bring your right foot toward you and strap the ball of your right foot. Lift your right leg, straighten your knee, and flex your toes toward you. Try to straighten both knees by lengthening your hamstrings. Place both ends of the strap in the right hand and bring your right leg down toward your right shoulder. Keep pressing the foot of the extended leg into the wall. Soften your throat, neck, and shoulders.

Hold for 20 to 30 seconds, increasing the time as you progress. Bring the right leg back to center before bringing your foot back to the wall. Switch sides.

Cautions/Hints
If your inner thighs are very stiff, you can stay in this pose longer, and you will be more comfortable, if you place a rolled-up blanket or very thick book under your upper thigh.

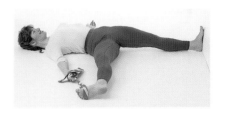

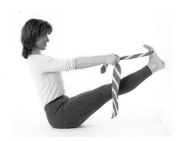

Abdominals

We all hate them; we all know we need to do them. Not only do abdominal exercises strengthen our stomach muscles, but they also strengthen our lower back muscles. So if your lower back is chronically painful and you are doing everything else you should be, add a few abs to your yoga routine.

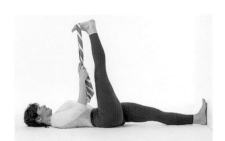

BOAT WITH STRAP

Sit facing a wall, 2 to 2½ feet from the wall. Place a necktie around the balls of your feet and place your heels on the wall about 2 feet from the floor. Lean back slightly so your torso forms a "V" with your legs. Lengthen your spine and lift your sternum. Firmly press your heels into the wall and press your thighs together.

Hold for 20 to 30 seconds, increasing the time as you progress. Release, rest, and try again.

Cautions/Hints
Keep lifting your lower back upward to prevent injury. If this is too easy, come away from the wall and firmly press your feet into the tie.

YOGA SIT-UPS

Lie on your back and with your knees bent, place your feet, hip distance apart, on a chair. Place your hands behind your head. Come up and try to touch your knees with your elbows. Only bring your back halfway to the floor after touching your elbows to your knees.

Do as many sit-ups as you can, increasing the number each time you practice.

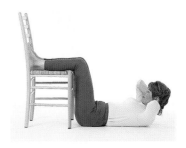

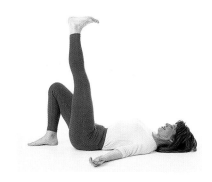

YOGA SIT-UPS 2

Lie on your back and place your calves on a chair. Place your right foot on your left knee. Place your hands behind your head, sit up, and bring your left elbow to your right knee. Only bring your back halfway to the floor after touching the elbow to the knee.

Do as many sit-ups on this side as you can, then switch the foot and knee position and bring your right elbow to your left knee. Increase the number of sit-ups each time you practice.

LEG LIFTS

Lie on your back with both legs extended straight in front of you. Place your hands underneath your hips. Bend your right knee and place the sole of your right foot as close to your hips as possible. Bring your left leg in toward your chest and then extend it straight out. Lift your leg straight up and then slowly bring it toward the floor. Hold your leg 2 to 3 inches from the floor for several seconds. Repeat several times and then switch sides.

Cautions/Hints
As you progress, you can lift both legs at once.

Twists

Twists open the chest, detoxify the body, "massage" the internal organs, and stretch the spine, giving it more flexibility.

Twists are good poses to do if you feel depressed, anxious, or fearful. The twists help "wring" the bad feelings out of your body, allowing you to face your fears or anxieties more easily and, most important, to get rid of them! If you use twists for this purpose, end the routine with a Passive Backbend (page 84) and Head to Chair Pose (page 80).

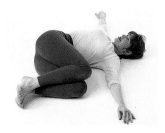

FEET ON THE FLOOR TWIST

Lie on your back with your knees bent and your feet on the floor near your hips. Extend your arms out to the side. With your legs and feet together, bring your legs to your left side. Keep your arms and shoulders on the floor.

Hold for 30 to 45 seconds. Come back to center and twist to the right.

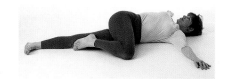

FOOT ON KNEE TWIST

Lie on your back, legs straight, feet flexed toward you. Extend your arms to your sides. Place your right foot on your left knee. Bring your right knee down to the left side. Continue extending your left leg and flex that foot toward you. Keep your head straight, looking at the ceiling. Keep your right shoulder as close to the floor as possible. It is better to keep your shoulder on the floor than to get your knee on the floor. Hold for 30 to 45 seconds. Come back to center and change sides.

CHAIR TWIST 1

Sit on the *edge* of your chair with your left side facing the back of the chair. Your feet and knees are together and need to stay that way throughout the pose. Place your hands on the chair as shown. On an inhalation straighten your spine, lifting from the very bottom of your spine. Descend your shoulders as you lift your rib cage. On an exhalation, twist toward the chair, twisting from the very bottom of your spine. Keep your face aligned with your chest. While twisting to the left, push with your right hand and pull with your left hand. Repeat the inhalation/straighten, exhalation/twist routine several times. Keep your throat, neck, and shoulders relaxed.

Release and switch sides. When twisting to the right, push with your left hand and pull with your right.

Cautions/Hints
For this pose and for Chair Twist 2, if your knees start to separate, press the leg that has moved back toward the one that hasn't moved.

CHAIR TWIST 2

Sit in the *middle* of your chair with your left side facing the back of the chair. Your feet and knees are together and need to stay that way throughout the pose. Place your hands on the chair as shown. On an inhalation straighten your spine, lifting from the very bottom of your spine. On an exhalation, twist toward the chair, twisting from the very bottom of your spine. Keep your face aligned with your chest. While twisting to the left, push with your right hand and pull with your left hand. Repeat the inhalation/straighten, exhalation/twist routine several times. Keep your neck, throat, and shoulders relaxed.

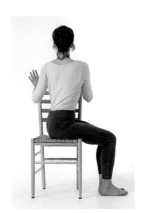

Release and switch sides so your right side is facing the chair. When twisting to the right, push with your left hand and pull with your right.

Cautions/Hints
When sitting in the middle of the chair seat, you will feel the twist more intensely in a different part of your spine.

Pre-Backbends

These poses are great to practice if you want to relieve tension in the neck, shoulders, and upper back. They also strengthen your legs and back, and give you a good stretch across your back, which helps keep the spine limber. These poses prepare us for doing backbends, which are definitely not for wimps!

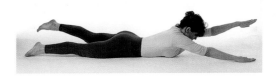

LOCUST VARIATION 1

Lie on your stomach with your legs straight and firm and with your arms straight out in front of you. Press your pubic bone firmly into the floor. Lift and extend your left arm and your left leg. Extend so much that you think your arms and legs will come out of their sockets. Keep your head in line with your spine, not tilted forward or backward.

Hold for 15 to 20 seconds, increasing the time as you progress. Release and then lift and extend your right arm and right leg. Repeat several times and rest before moving into the next pose.

Cautions/Hints
For this pose and the other two Locust poses, if you physically have the choice of extending more or lifting higher, extend more. Continually press your pubic bone into the floor to protect your lower back.

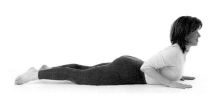

COBRA

Lie on your stomach and place your hands on the sides of your chest. Firmly press your pubic bone into the floor and keep your legs straight and firm. Raise your chest, curving your upper back inward, extending your chest outward, and lifting your sternum. Keep your lower rib cage on the floor. Your arms should be at the side of your torso. Your head is in line with your spine. Do not tilt your head backward — that will only give you a neckache!

Cautions/Hints
Continually press your pubic bone into the floor to help protect your lower back.

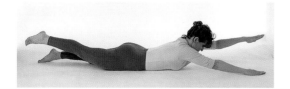

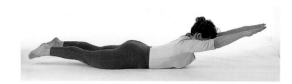

LOCUST VARIATION 2

Lie on your stomach with your legs straight and firm and with your arms straight out in front of you. Press your pubic bone firmly into the floor. Lift and extend your left arm and your right leg. Extend so much that you think your arms and legs will come out of their sockets. Keep your head in line with your spine, not tilted forward or backward. Hold for 15 to 20 seconds. Release, and lift and extend your right arm and your left leg.

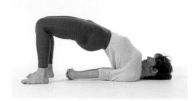

DESK

Lie on your back with your knees bent and your feet as close to your hips as possible. Place your feet so they are hip distance apart. Lift your hips, clasp your hands underneath your back, and roll your shoulders under. Lift your hips as high as possible. Roll your thighs inward. Keep lifting your hips!

Hold for 30 to 45 seconds, increasing the time as you progress. Rest, and try again.

Cautions/Hints

This pose is great for building lower back strength. But to do so, it is very important to keep your hips lifting as high as possible.

FULL LOCUST

Lie on your stomach with your legs straight and firm and with your arms straight out in front of you. Press your pubic bone into the floor. Lift and extend both arms and both legs. Extend so much that you think your arms and legs will come out of their sockets. Keep your head in line with your spine, not tilted forward or backward. Hold for 15 to 20 seconds. Release, rest with your cheek on your hands for a few moments, and try again.

Passive Backbends

Passive backbends are among yoga's greatest gifts. The only effort involved is getting your props right. These poses relax the body, the mind, and the emotions. Your chest expands, allowing you to take in more oxygen. More oxygen simply makes us feel more alive!

If you are emotionally upset, these poses allow the pain, fear, or heartache to surface and release. In other words, passive backbends harmonize the spirit.

If you are tired, try these poses instead of a nap. They allow you to rest on a very deep level and thus, will increase your energy. If you are wide awake at 2 in the morning and cannot get back to sleep, try one or two of these in bed. Your mind will quiet, allowing sleep to return.

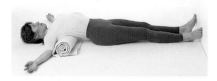

SUPPORTED CHEST OPENER

Roll up a blanket or towel and place it under your upper middle back, behind the sternum. If you like, you can use a pillow or folded blanket under your head. Cover your eyes and relax.

Cautions/Hints

Try various heights of blanket or towel to determine what works for your body. You may prefer a thin roll. A thicker roll may require a pillow or folded blanket under your head. Experiment!

PASSIVE BACKBEND SERIES

Roll up a blanket or two. Place the roll directly behind your sternum and lie over it. Rest for a few moments to determine if you like the height or not. If necessary, adjust to a height you prefer. You can also try placing folded blankets under your head, neck, and shoulders to determine if that is more comfortable.

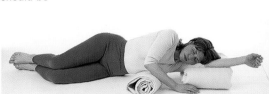

Sit in front of your blanket setup, with 2 neckties that are knotted together on one end. Come into Bound Angle Pose:

- Bring the soles of your feet together.

- Place the ties around your lower back, over the top of your right thigh and calf, around the outside of your feet, and over the top of your left thigh and calf. Knot the neckties with the knot falling between your calf and thigh. The ties should be taut but not so tight that you will have no mobility when you lie down.

- Lie back over your blanket roll, so the roll is directly behind your sternum.

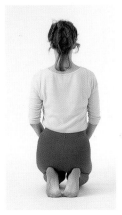

- If your lower back hurts, place a thick book under your feet.

- If you feel discomfort in your thighs or knees, place a pillow or rolled-up blanket under the middle of your thigh.

- Then lie here as long as you like. I can easily stay in this pose for 20 to 30 minutes, often falling asleep. When you feel finished with this pose, with as little disturbance to your body as possible, undo the ties and extend your legs. You are still in the basic reclining backbend, but now your legs are straight. Stay in this pose as long as you like.

- When you are ready, roll over to your left side. Stay there until you are ready to roll over to your right side. You may need an extra blanket on hand for your head. Or you can use your arm as an extra lift.

- Slowly come out of the sequence at any point you like.

Feet Poses

If your feet have never been stretched or regularly massaged, these poses could initially be quite uncomfortable, but you will love the benefits. As you advance in your practice, you will actually enjoy the poses and will want to spend more time in them. Your feet will soon feel terrific!

FEET SITTING

Kneel with your legs, feet, and ankles together. Curl your toes under — making sure you get the little ones, too — and sit back on your heels. To decrease the intensity, keep your fingers on the floor. To intensify the stretch, tie a necktie around your ankles to hold them together. Hold for 15 to 20 seconds, increasing the time as you become more comfortable in the pose. Release, rest, and try again.

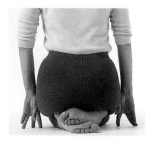

FOOT IN ARCH STRETCH

Kneel down, torso up and feet extended so that the tops of the feet are on the floor and the toes are extended naturally. Place the front top half of your right foot into the arch of your left foot. Then sit back on your heels. This stretch will massage your left foot, stretch your left ankle, and stretch the top of your right foot and ankle.

This pose is bound to be a little awkward at first, so initially stay in this pose for 20 to 30 seconds and then switch sides, placing your top left foot into the arch of your right foot.

Cautions/Hints
As you progress in this pose, you can try placing your top foot on various parts of your bottom foot, thus massaging your entire foot.

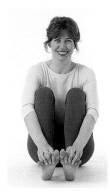

FINGERS BETWEEN TOES

This is very easy to do! While sitting, simply intertwine your fingers between your toes. It doesn't matter if you approach the toes from the front of the foot or from the soles. To amplify the stretch, you may want to flex your ankle, or curl your toes toward the front of your ankle.

You can do these toe stretches for whatever amount of time you like, but at a minimum, hold the poses for at least a minute. If your feet are particularly sore, do this several times.

Standing Poses

Standing poses are the foundation poses. They build leg strength, and more important, they build lower back strength. The lower back muscles are the body's weakest muscles, yet they carry the heaviest load. I have read statistics stating that 90 percent of all adults have lower back pain. If you suffer from lower back pain, regular practice of these poses can start giving you immediate relief.

Standing poses are vigorous and are good to do if you need extra energy — if you are a little sleepy in the morning or at the end of the day when your work is not yet done.

In addition to strengthening your body, standing poses also strengthen your spirit. This makes perfect sense — if you fortify the foundation of your body (feet, legs, and lower back), your spirit will feel empowered! It is no mistake that three of the standing poses are named "Warrior Pose." Sometimes we need to be warriors just to get through the trials of life. So if you need some extra vigor, power, or courage in your life, do the standing poses. And if you need a lot of extra bolstering, do each pose several times!

In each of the following poses, I give the instruction of lifting your thighs and rolling them either inward or outward. It may take some time for your thighs to actually do this. To lift the thigh is simply to engage the quadriceps muscles, bringing them up toward the abdomen. Some people say you are contracting the knee, but in reality you are contracting the quadriceps muscles *without* locking the knee joint. Call it what you want, just make sure you practice it.

You can practice rolling your thighs inward and outward with your hands. Manually roll your thighs, then release as you continue with the rest of the pose. This way your body can learn what the "outward-rolling" or "inward-rolling" feeling is. Continue practicing, you will get it! And when you do, you will notice a tremendous feeling of freedom in your lower back.

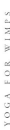

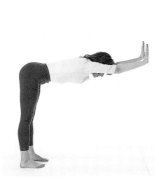
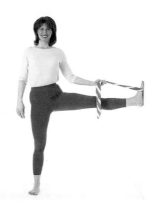
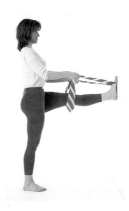

RIGHT ANGLE POSE

Stand close to the wall, facing it. Place your hands on the wall at waist height. Make sure that your hands are shoulder width apart, and firmly planted on the wall. Fingers are spread and "alive with energy." Your feet are 1) directly under your hips, 2) hip width apart, and 3) firmly planted on the floor. Walk your feet back until your body is perpendicular to the wall (or parallel to the floor) and your legs are at a right angle to your torso. Your arms and legs should be completely straight, or at least working on becoming straight. Lift your quadriceps muscles and roll your thigh muscles inward. Extend your spine as much as possible. Keep pressing your hands into the wall. Press as though you are trying to push the wall over! Press the front of your thighs to the back of your thighs. (Imagine this until you get it!)

Hold for 30 to 45 seconds, increasing the time as you progress. Release the pose by stepping toward the wall.

Cautions/Hints
Extend your spine as much as you can in this pose, as though your spine were made of those "pop beads" we used to play with as kids. Imagine that the beads, or your vertebrae, are fully extended.

LEG-TO-CHAIR, TABLE, OR WALL POSE — SIDE ANGLE

Stand with your left side facing the table, chair, or wall — a leg's distance away. Stand with your feet together, your weight evenly distributed to both legs. Lift your quadriceps muscles. Lengthen your lower back and lift your sternum. Relax your throat, neck, and shoulders. Shift your weight to your right leg, turn your left foot outward, and place the strap around the ball of your foot. Then lift your left leg and place your heel on the table or chair, or the sole of your foot on the wall. Firmly press your standing foot into the floor. If you are using a chair or a table, flex your left foot toward you. Continue to check your posture in the pose.

Initially hold this pose for 20 to 30 seconds, increasing the time as you progress. Release and switch sides.

Cautions/Hints
Ideally, when lifted, your leg should be aligned with your hip. If this is not possible, start with the prop that is easiest for you — a chair or table that is shorter than your hip crease.

LEG-TO-CHAIR, TABLE, OR WALL POSE — FRONT ANGLE

Stand facing a table, a chair, or a wall — a leg's distance away. Stand with your feet together, your weight evenly distributed. Lift your quadriceps muscles. Lengthen your lower back and lift your sternum. Shift your weight to your right leg, lift your left leg, and place the strap around the ball of your foot. Then place the heel of your left leg on the table or chair, or the sole of your foot on the wall. Where you place your foot depends on your flexibility. Hold one side of the tie in each hand. Press the front of the thighs to the back of the thighs and check your posture in the pose. Try to keep the toes of the standing foot facing the prop — not turned outward — and keep the front hipbones as even as possible.

Initially hold this pose for 20 to 30 seconds, increasing the time as you progress. Release and switch sides.

Cautions/Hints
Ideally, when lifted, your leg should be aligned with your hip. If this is not possible, start with the prop that is easiest for you — a chair or table that is shorter than your hip crease.

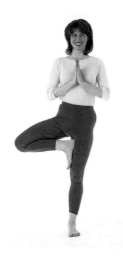

TREE POSE

Stand with either your right or left side facing the wall, feet together. Lengthen your lower back and lift your sternum. Lift your quadriceps muscles and roll your thighs outward. Bend whichever leg faces the wall so your knee is on the wall and your foot is on your inner thigh. Place your tie around your shin if you need help keeping your leg in place. Press your foot into your thigh and your thigh into your foot.

Hold for 20 to 30 seconds, increasing the time as you progress. Release and switch sides.

Cautions/Hints
When you no longer need the tie or the wall, practice the pose in the middle of the room and place your hands, in prayer position, at your heart.

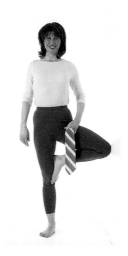

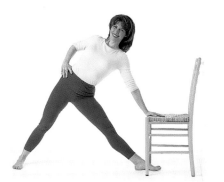
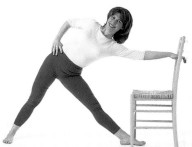

TRIANGLE POSE

Place the back of your chair at the wall. Stand with your left side facing the chair seat. Your feet are 2½ to 3 feet apart. Place the toes of your left foot under the chair seat, aligning the heel of your left foot with the arch of your right foot. Lift your quadriceps muscles and turn your thigh muscles outward. Lengthen your lower back and lift your sternum. Extend your arms outward, shoulder height, palms facing downward, and elbows straight. From the hip crease, laterally lean toward the chair. Place your left hand on the chair, either on the seat or on the chair back, and place your right hand on your hip. Keep your head aligned with your spine, and look forward.

Hold for 20 to 30 seconds, increasing the time as you progress. Release and switch sides.

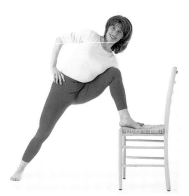

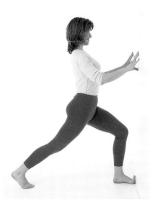

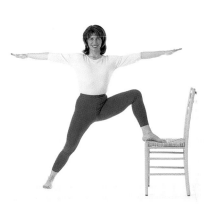

SIDE ANGLE POSE

Place the back of your chair at the wall. Stand with your left side facing the chair. Your feet are 2½ to 3 feet apart. Place your left foot on the chair seat, aligning the heel of your left foot with the arch of your right foot. Lift your quadriceps muscles and turn your thigh muscles outward. Lengthen your lower back and lift your sternum. Extend your arms outward, shoulder height, palms facing downward, and elbows straight. Bend the left knee into a right angle. Moving from the hip crease, extend the side of your torso over your thigh. Rest your elbow on your knee or your hand on the chair seat. Place your right hand on your hip. Align your torso and legs by moving your chest up and back. Look forward.

Hold for 20 to 30 seconds, increasing the time as you progress. Release and switch sides.

Cautions/Hints
As you progress in this pose, you can lower the height of your prop. Use a step or some stacked books. Eventually you will have the forward foot on the floor. Once you are on the floor, place the back foot at the wall and separate your feet by 4 to 4½ feet.

WARRIOR I

Stand facing a wall, 2½ to 3½ feet from the wall; legs are hip distance apart. Extend your left leg forward to the wall and place your toes at the wall. Lengthen your lower back and lift your sternum. Place your hands on the wall about waist height. Relax your throat, neck, and shoulders. Lift your quadriceps muscles and turn your back thigh inward and your forward thigh outward. Keeping your back leg as straight as possible (your heel can be lifted) and your front hipbones even, slowly bend your front knee toward the wall. With the help of the wall, steady your pose. Keep lifting your chest. Hold for 20 to 30 seconds, release, and do the pose with your right leg forward.

Cautions/Hints
As you become more proficient in the pose, allow the back leg to be farther back and bend your forward knee into a right angle. However, there is no hurry to get there!

WARRIOR II

Place the back of your chair at the wall. Stand with your left side facing the front of the chair, your feet 2½ to 3 feet apart. Place your left foot on the chair seat. Align the heel of the forward foot with the arch of the back foot. Lift your quadriceps and roll your thighs outward. Lengthen your lower back and lift your sternum. Extend your arms, shoulder height, palms facing downward. Relax your throat, neck, and shoulders. Slowly bend your left knee into a right angle. Continue to keep your back leg straight and your back foot pressing into the floor. Look straight ahead or out over the forward hand.

Hold for 20 to 30 seconds, increasing the time as you progress. Release and switch sides.

Cautions/Hints
As you progress in this pose, you can lower the height of your prop. Use a step or some stacked books. Eventually you will have the forward foot on the floor. Once you are on the floor, place the back foot at the wall and separate your feet by 4 to 4½ feet.

WARRIOR III

The first part of this pose is Right Angle Pose (page 87). Stand close to the wall, facing it. Your legs are hip width apart. Place your hands on the wall at waist height. Your hands are shoulder distance apart. Walk your feet back until your body is perpendicular to the wall and your legs are at a right angle to your torso. Plant your feet firmly on the floor and roll your thighs inward. Straighten your arms and legs. Firmly press your hands into the wall, as though you are going to topple it. Extend your spine as much as you can in this pose. Then, shift your weight to the left leg. Lift your right leg so it is parallel to the floor and in line with your hips, i.e., not above and not below the hips. However, below the hips is better than above the hips! Try to keep the front hipbones even. (Both of these actions will take lots of practice, so don't get discouraged!) Extend your leg as much as you can and flex your toes toward you. Continue to lengthen your arms, spine, and legs. Keep pressing your hands into the wall as though you want to knock it over.

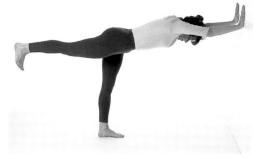

Hold for 15 to 20 seconds, increasing the time as you progress. Release and switch sides.

Cautions/Hints

Make sure you extend your spine and leg to your absolute maximum. Keep the front hipbones even — or at least as even as you can. As shown in Slaying the Stress Monster (on page 60), you can have someone help you keep your leg straight and your hipbones even.

Standing Forward Bends

These forward bends will stretch your inner thigh muscles, hamstrings, hips, and lower back, restoring flexibility and bringing relief to that nagging back pain.

In some of these poses, you allow your back to round. But in most of them, your back needs to be straight. If you do the action correctly, you will build strength in your lower back muscles. The correct action, unless stated otherwise, is to lengthen your lower back and lift your sternum. As you bend from the hip crease, consciously elongate your back. Lifting your sternum helps keep your upper back straight.

Usually in standing forward bends you lift your quadriceps muscles and roll your thighs inward. Review the instructions for practicing these moves in the Standing Poses section (page 86).

STANDING FORWARD BEND 1

Stand in front of the chair seat, a leg's distance away, and place your left heel on the chair seat. Flex your toes toward you and place a tie around the ball of your foot. Lift your quadriceps and roll your thighs inward. The toes of your standing leg face the chair. Lengthen your lower back and lift your sternum. Relax your throat, neck, and shoulders. From the hip crease, bend forward. Only move as far forward as you can with your back straight.

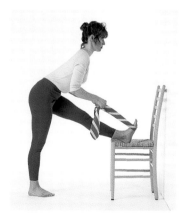

Hold for 30 to 45 seconds, increasing the time as you progress. Release and switch sides.

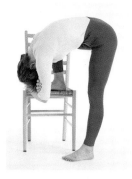
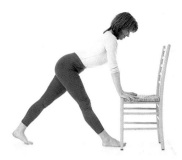
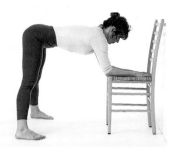

STANDING FORWARD BEND 2

Stand with your feet separated about 12 inches and your right side touching the chair seat. Lift your right leg and place your foot on the chair seat. Roll the thigh muscles of the lifted leg outward. Lift the quadriceps muscles of the standing leg. From the hip crease, lean forward — rounding your back. You can relax in the pose by clasping your elbows. Or you can work in the pose by pulling on the chair seat or chair legs. Completely drop your head and relax your neck. Breathe deeply into your lower back and with each exhalation allow your entire body to relax a little more.

Hold as long as you like, increasing the time as you progress. Release and switch sides.

Cautions/Hints
If you are not comfortable in this pose, try the Chair Lower Back Stretch on page 79 instead.

STANDING HAMSTRING STRETCH

Stand facing your chair. Place your right foot halfway under the chair seat and your back foot 3 to 3½ feet from your front foot. Lengthen your lower back and lift your sternum. Relax your throat, neck, and shoulders. From the hip crease, bend toward the chair — continually straightening your back. Place your hands on the chair back or the chair seat. As you gain flexibility, place your forearms on the chair seat, but only do this if you can keep your back straight. Make sure your head is in line with your spine.

Hold for 30 to 45 seconds, increasing the time as you progress. Release and switch sides.

STANDING WIDE ANGLE POSE

Place the chair back at the wall. Stand facing the chair, 2 feet from the chair seat, with your feet 2½ to 3 feet wide. Lift your quadriceps muscles and roll your thighs inward. Lengthen your lower back and lift your sternum. From the hip crease, bend toward the chair — continually straightening your back. Place your hands on the chair back or the chair seat. As you gain flexibility, place your forearms on the chair seat, but only do this if you can keep your back straight.

Hold for 30 to 45 seconds, increasing the time as you progress.

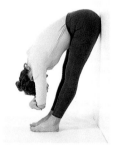

WALL HANG

Stand with your feet 12 to 18 inches from the wall and your buttocks on the wall. Your feet are hip distance apart. With your hands, walk your buttocks up the wall a little. Roll your thighs inward. From the hip crease, bend forward. Initially you can round your back, but as you progress your back will straighten. Try two positions in this pose. First, keep your knees straight with your quadriceps lifted and your thighs rolling inward. Drop your head completely, soften your neck, and hold your elbows. Hold this first pose for 30 seconds. Then bend your knees to get more release in your lower back. Hold this second pose as long as you like. Come up slowly on an inhalation.

Cautions/Hints
If this pose is not comfortable for you, do the Chair Lower Back Stretch on page 79.

Calves and Quads

Often people forget to stretch two important areas — calves and quadriceps. When you stretch these areas you increase flexibility *and* help prevent injuries.

The calf stretches are especially intense for women who wear high heels and for runners and swimmers. If you fall into one of these categories, do these poses several times a week. These poses are good to practice with the foot stretches in Oh My Aching Feet (pages 52–55).

Stretching the quadriceps muscles lengthens the abdominal muscles and the psoas muscles, which connect the spine, pelvis, hip joints, and thighs. If these muscles are tight, your posture can be negatively affected and can lead to lower back pain. Be sure to include quad stretches in your routine.

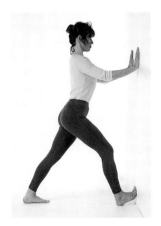

CALF STRETCH 1

Stand facing the wall, about two feet from the wall. Place your hands on the wall at shoulder height. Bring your right foot to the wall, placing the ball of the foot up the wall. The heel of the back foot can lift. You should immediately feel a stretch along the forward calf muscles. If you want a more intense stretch, lean your body into the wall, resting your chest and head on the wall if you wish.

Hold as long as you can — 15 seconds if your calves are very tight — or 45 to 60 seconds if the stretch feels good. Release and switch sides. Repeat several times.

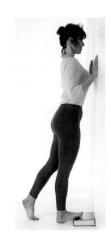

CALF STRETCH 2

Place a dictionary or any other thick book against the wall, with the spine of the book facing outward. Place the ball of your right foot on the book. Then, simply allow your heel to come back down to the floor. Use the wall or a chair for balance. To intensify the stretch, use a thicker book or a step.

Hold as long as you can — 15 seconds if your calves are very tight — or 45 to 60 seconds if the stretch feels good. Release and switch sides. Repeat several times.

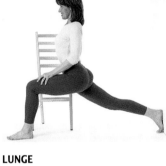

LUNGE

Kneel with the soles of your feet on the wall. Bring your left leg forward so your thigh and calf are just a little wider than a right angle (approximately a 120-degree angle). Hold onto the chair for support if needed. Sink your hips toward the floor and then straighten your back knee. Keeping the back leg straight, sink your hips again. Try to keep your front hipbones even. Continue to press your back heel into the wall.

Hold for 20 to 30 seconds, increasing the time as you progress. Release and switch sides.

Cautions/Hints
It is recommended that you first use a chair for the quad stretches. When you no longer need the chair for balance, come into the poses with your torso erect and after a few moments, bring your hands to the floor.

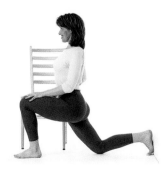

QUADRICEPS STRETCH

Kneel with the soles of your feet on the wall. Bring your left leg forward so your thigh and calf are just a little wider than a right angle (approximately a 120-degree angle). Keeping your right knee on the floor and your right foot pressing into the wall, start to sink your hips toward the floor. Try to keep your front hipbones even.

Hold the pose for 20 to 30 seconds, increasing the time as you progress. Release and switch sides.

Cautions/Hints
For variation, place the top of your right foot on the floor and press it into the floor.

Arm Stretches

This section includes several poses that you can do while you're walking around or in a seated pose. Some of the poses require a chair. If you like, you can do all of these poses as a routine. The arm stretches will release tension in your upper back, shoulders, and neck. As your neck and shoulders relax, you will find that headaches go away, and if you have sinus problems, you will notice some improvement.

If you feel energized after doing these poses, try some of the poses from the Building Upper Body Strength section that follows.

Reminder: In all of these poses, keep your throat, neck, and shoulders relaxed. Breathe into these areas as you work, so you can experience as much softening as possible in the poses.

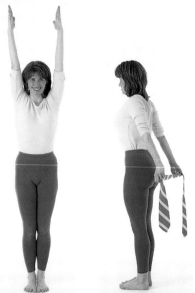

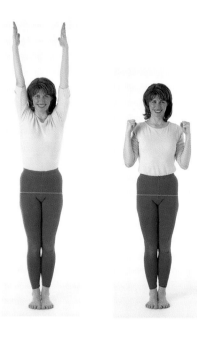

ARM STRETCH 1

Stretch your arms straight overhead, palms facing each other. Stretch as though you are stretching from your hips, not just from your shoulders. Be sure to keep your neck and shoulders relaxed as you do this. Hold for 30 to 45 seconds, release, and repeat.

ARM STRETCH 2

Bring your arms behind your back, holding a tie with your hands. Lift your arms only as high as you can keep your sternum lifted.

As you gain flexibility, move your hands closer on the tie. Or forget the tie and interlock your fingers. Hold for 30 to 45 seconds, release, relax for a moment, and repeat.

ARM STRETCH 3

Interlock your fingers and extend your arms straight in front of you. Slowly lift your arms overhead. Stretch as though you are stretching all the way from your lower back. Hold for 30 to 45 seconds, release, relax for a moment, and try again.

THE BEST ARM EXTENSIONS

While extending your arms over your head, palms facing each other, inhale as deeply as you can. When you have reached your full extension, make a fist. Exhale quickly and bend your elbows — bringing your fists to your shoulders and your upper arms to the sides of your chest.

Do this 8 or 10 times, rest, and repeat another series of 8 or 10.

Cautions/Hints
Take deep, exaggerated breaths, exhaling forcefully. Be sure your neck is relaxed. This is a particularly powerful technique and it is sure to invigorate you.

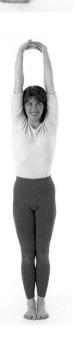

UPWARD ARM STRETCH (far left)

Sit near the edge of the chair seat, facing the wall. Your knees can touch the wall. Place your hands as high on the wall as possible. Then walk your fingers up the wall, stretching as though you are stretching from your lower back. Broaden your shoulders by separating your shoulder blades. Keep your neck and throat soft. Don't tense your shoulders, just lift them. Once you think your fingers are as high as they can be, walk them a little higher.

Release, rest for a few moments, and try again.

Cautions/Hints
This pose is also great for relieving tension in the lower back, if you're careful to stretch from the lower back.

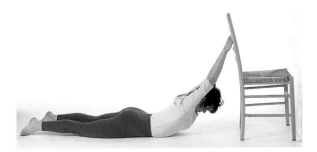

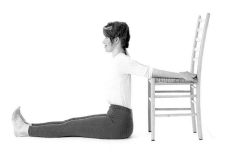

FORWARD ARM STRETCH

Lie on your stomach, facing the back of the chair. Place your body so that when you extend your arms, your wrists are aligned with the chair legs that are closest to you. Reach up with both hands and grasp the chair at the highest place you possibly can. If the highest place for you is the top of the chair, great! If not, place your hands as high up on the sides as possible, or on the chair seat. When you place your hands on the chair, your upper torso should come up from the floor, but not your stomach. Press your pubic bone into the floor for stability. Scoot the chair forward until your elbows are straight and the front chair legs are lifted. Broaden your shoulders by separating your shoulder blades. Keep your neck relaxed and your head in line with your arms. Start moving the front legs of the chair back toward the floor. You will feel your chest expanding, and your arms and shoulders extending.

Hold as long as you like. Release, relax with your cheek on your hands, and try again.

BACKWARD ARM STRETCH

Sit comfortably in front of your chair seat. Lengthen your spine and lift your sternum. Reach back and grasp the sides of the chair at whatever height is comfortable for you. If you are a little more flexible, you can place your hands on the back of the chair seat. Roll your shoulders forward and down. Continue to lift your sternum. Your neck and throat are relaxed.

Hold as long as you can, rest, and repeat.

Building Upper Body Strength

You may find these poses to be quite difficult, even if you already have a strong upper body. These poses use muscles that are not normally used in "western" exercises. They build strength and flexibility in the arms, shoulders, and upper back. Regular practice can help straighten a curved spine in the upper back, and improve posture quickly.

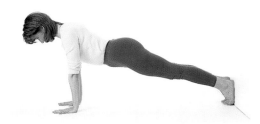

PLANK POSE

Kneel on all fours with your feet at the wall and your arms at a 120-degree angle to your torso (i.e., slightly more than a right angle). Make sure your fingers are spread and your hands are firmly pressing into the floor. Shift your weight over your hands. Then curl your toes under and straighten your arms and knees, so your body resembles a plank or board. Draw your arm muscles and your shoulders toward the ceiling. Keep your lower back and lower abdomen moving in toward each other. Extend your legs, pushing your feet into the wall. Keep your head in line with your spine.

Hold this pose for 10 to 15 seconds, increasing the time as you progress.

Cautions/Hints

If your wrists hurt in this pose, place a rolled-up towel under the heel of your hands. This way, the heel of your palm is on the towel and your fingers are on the floor. It is very important to keep drawing your arm muscles and your shoulders toward the ceiling as much as possible while pressing your feet into the wall as much as you can.

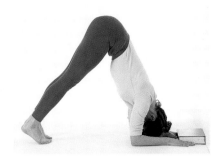

PRE-ELBOW BALANCE

Place a dictionary against the wall, with the spine of the book facing you. Kneel down, placing your thumbs in front of the book and your index fingers on the side. Your forearms are on the floor. Keeping your forearms on the floor, come up on your toes. Straighten your knees if you can and walk in toward the wall. Keep lifting your shoulders — to your absolute maximum — and walk in a little more. Allow your head to hang toward the floor without placing it on the floor.

If your knees don't completely straighten, don't force them. Hold the pose for a few seconds (or longer if you like), increasing the time as you progress. Rest in Child's Pose (below) for a few moments and try again.

Cautions/Hints

To help keep your elbows properly placed, tie an old necktie an inch above your elbows and adjust the tightness so that your elbows are aligned with your shoulders. Hint for this pose and the next one: To help straighten your upper back and keep your shoulders lifted, have a friend lean against the wall with bent knees. Walk into your friend's knees (they should be at or near your shoulder blades). When your friend releases, try to keep your back as straight as it was and your shoulders lifted as much as they were when your friend was helping you. See Slaying the Stress Monster on page 58 for photographic detail.

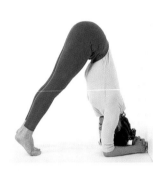

PRE-HEADSTAND

Interlock your fingers, kneel down, and place the back of your hands against the wall and your forearms on the floor. Your elbows are directly under your shoulders. Come up on your toes, lifting your buttocks toward the ceiling. If you can, straighten your knees. Walk in toward the wall, lifting your shoulders continuously. Allow your head to hang down. Keep lifting your shoulders to your absolute maximum!

Hold the pose for a few seconds (or longer if you like), increasing the time as you progress. Rest in Child's Pose (below) for a few moments and try again.

Cautions/Hints

You don't need any props for this pose unless you find that your arms slip or are uncomfortable. If you have either problem, place a blanket under your arms.

Resting Poses

If you are tired, catching a cold, or just want to pamper yourself, practice this series as presented. These poses help release and soften the neck, shoulders, and back — increasing flexibility and simply making you feel better.

When you are practicing more strenuous poses, rest in one of these postures from time to time. And, as always, end your practice with a resting pose. But if you have time, do more than one — you'll be glad you did!

CHILD'S POSE

From a kneeling position, widen your thighs, place your buttocks on your heels, and bring your torso toward the floor. Rest your forehead on the floor, a book, or a blanket. If your body doesn't reach your heels, place a folded blanket or two on your feet. Rest with your arms in front of you or beside you. Breathe into your lower back and with each exhalation, allow your body to soften and relax just a little bit more.

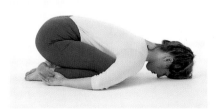

Cautions/Hints

If you have an injured knee, or if this is not comfortable for any reason, practice the Chair Lower Back Stretch instead (see page 79).

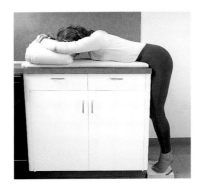

KITCHEN COUNTER POSE

Fold or roll up some blankets or towels and place them on the kitchen counter. Lean over the counter from the hip crease, if possible, and place your torso on the roll-up. If you are too short for the kitchen counter, either stand on some thick books or place your roll-up on a long credenza or bureau. If your counter is short, add a roll-up under your torso. If your neck is uncomfortable, fold an extra blanket or towel and place it under your forehead. Lie here as long as you like, completely relaxing with each exhalation.

Cautions/Hints
If your upper back naturally rounds outward, this pose may not be comfortable.

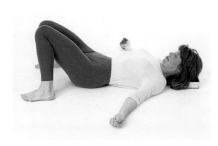

BOOK SUPPORT

Place a dictionary or similar sized book on the floor. Lie on your back, placing your head on the book with your knees bent and together, and your feet wider than hip distance apart.

Cautions/Hints
If this is not comfortable, try a thinner book. If that doesn't work, try a thicker one. For deeper relaxation, place a small towel or your yoga tie over your eyes.

CHAIR CORPSE POSE

Lie on the floor and place your calves on the chair seat. You may want to cover yourself with a blanket, put earplugs in your ears, and place a small towel or your yoga tie over your eyes. This way you can melt into the pose without any noise or light pollution. Once you are in the pose, allow each exhalation to relax your body and quiet your mind just a little bit more. If you are like me, you will fall asleep in this pose and awaken naturally. When you are ready to get up, bring your knees to your chest and stay there for a few moments. Roll over to your right side. Keeping your neck completely soft, use your hand and elbow to push yourself up into a seated position. Sit for a few moments, enjoying your newly found relaxation.

Cautions/Hints
If your neck is not completely comfortable, place a pillow or folded blanket under your head.

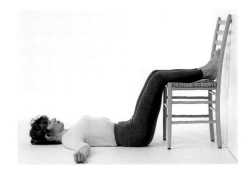

Miscellaneous Poses

Here you will find various poses that don't fit into a specific category.

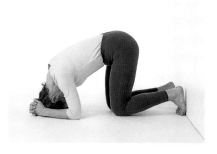

HEAD ROLL

Kneel on all fours and place your head on the floor. Slowly roll your head forward toward your forehead and then backward to the very top of your head. Repeat this movement several times.

Cautions/Hints

This should be done on a carpeted floor or using a thick towel or blanket. This pose will activate the pressure points on the top of your head and help ease head and neck pain.

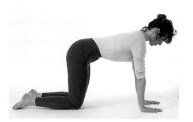

TABLE

Kneel on all fours. Extend your spine and lift your shoulders.

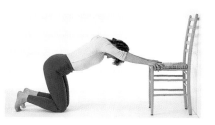

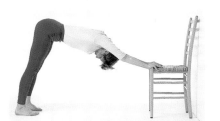

DOWNWARD FACING DOG

Place the back of the chair against the wall. Kneel on all fours, with your knees 2 to 2½ feet from the chair and your toes curled under. Place your hands on the edge of the chair. Curve your lower back inward and move your buttocks up toward the ceiling. Come up on your toes, keeping your buttocks high and angling your torso downward. Extend your arms and torso as much as possible. Lift your quadriceps muscles and roll your thighs inward. Try to straighten your knees. On each inhalation, lengthen your arms and torso. On each exhalation, move the front of your thighs to the back of your thighs.

Hold for 30 to 45 seconds, increasing the time as you progress in the pose. Release, rest in Child's Pose (page 94), and try again.

Cautions/Hints

Keep moving the front of your thighs toward the back of your thighs. Have a friend pull the top of your thighs backward, holding them there for a few moments, so you know how great the pose will feel when done properly. (See Slaying the Stress Monster on page 56 for photographic detail.) This will take the weight off your arms. As you become more proficient in this pose, you can start to use lower props. For example, you can use a step or thick books until you can do the pose with your hands on the floor.

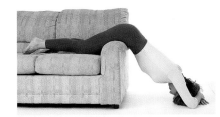

HANGING OFF THE COUCH

Climb on the couch and place your hip crease at the edge of the arm. Lean over toward the floor, holding your elbows if you like. Just hang there as long as you like, relaxing completely and allowing the tension to melt away.

Cautions/Hints

If your couch arm is short for your height, try leaning over the back of the couch — but just in case, you may want someone to hold onto your legs. This is a wonderful pose. It quickly releases tension in the lower back.

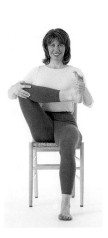

ROCK THE BABY

Sit in the chair, keeping your back as straight as possible. Bring your right leg up, close to your chest. Place your right foot in your left hand and your right knee in your right hand. Bring your calf parallel to the floor and even with your chest, if possible. Move your leg from side to side, as though you are rocking a baby.

Cautions/Hints

If you cannot get your calf even with your chest, don't worry, that will come with practice. Keep lengthening your lower back and lifting your sternum.

If you find this pose easy, place your foot and knee in the crook of each elbow.

A Final Word

Yoga transforms our lives in many ways. We all experience pain and suffering — they are part of life. We get sick or injured, our loved ones die, we are laid off from our jobs, our spouses leave us — the list can go on and on. We have no control over many of the events that cause our suffering. Furthermore, we all experience pain that is a reflection of our conditioning — the result of parenting, peer response, schooling, and cultural values. And because we have pain, we either search for some meaning to our lives or we search for something meaningful.

What is meaningful to each of us varies, and may change at different stages of our lives. But generally the things we all want most are love and happiness. The first benefit of yoga is that we start to feel more alive, more connected to our bodies. And as we continue our yoga practice, other benefits manifest. We find both significance in and acceptance of life's mysteries; we find more love, joy, and purpose.

Yoga helps us live in a new way: it returns us to a state of wholeness. Many of us live "in our heads." The danger in this is that the mind tends to be critical and judgmental — of ourselves and others. Through yoga, our energy and focus come down through the body and our body's own intelligence awakens. Our hearts expand and our capacity for love increases.

We awaken to the inner love and joy that is our true nature. Many people think that they are "in love" or that they "experience love," but the truth is that we are love. Our essence, the very core of our being, is love. And as we practice yoga, that essence grows. The loneliness that many of us feel, whether we have a special loved one in our lives or not, diminishes as we awaken to the only love that will permanently sustain us — our own essence of love. We begin to feel complete. Our apprehensions of ourselves and others fall away. We learn that life's inevitable sadnesses and difficulties can be soul expanding. Our compassion and our empathy broaden to encompass more and more people. We slowly find ourselves appreciating those we may have criticized in the past. As we break down the barriers that block us from our own inner love, we remove the barricades that prevent loving relationships with others. We begin to radiate love, joy, happiness, and inner harmony to those around us. And we soon find that the love we give to others is abundantly returned to us.

This book encourages uncovering our hidden potential. Somehow we all know, deep down inside, that love, joy, happiness, and inner harmony are our birthright. Through yoga, we can "return" to this natural state. Through yoga, life can be an adventure brimming with enthusiasm and joy!

About the Models

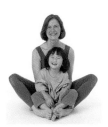

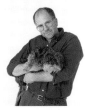

Sam Yoder has practiced meditation and carpentry for the past twenty years. He has practiced hatha yoga since we asked him to model for this book.

Nancy Crum Stechert, a former marathoner, came to yoga more than twenty years ago to stretch out after running. She pursued her study of yoga with B.K.S. Iyengar in India. Nancy founded the Colorado School of Yoga and the International Yoga School in Tokyo. She relies on yoga to make sure she doesn't wimp out on her most demanding roles as wife and mother of two.

Carol Kitching is a vision therapist living in Oregon with her family of four. See her if you can't read the fine print in this book.

Laura Washington is a naturopathic physician and founder of Art of Health, Inc., a medicinal tea company based in Portland, Oregon. Sleepy, grumpy, and dopey are all states she can remedy with her tonics. She's working on wimpy.

Lubosh Cech rode night trains and crossed under barbed wire to escape from his native Czechoslovakia in 1983. Since his emigration to the United States he has worked as a designer, photographer, and art director. Lubosh designed this book, right down to the very page you are reading now. If you like it, thank him.

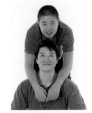

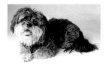

Shizeng Yang lived the first part of his life in China, where he studied massage and played professional handball. After moving to the United States, he served as a professor at the Oregon College of Oriental Medicine. Shizeng currently practices the ancient art of Tui Na massage and the even more ancient art of raising a teenage son, Simon.

Albert Norbu has pursued a career of security work from a very early age. Albert has gained a reputation as an expert Polaroid lighting checker and has availed his services on several publishing projects.

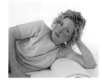

Katie Southworth helps run New Traditions in Health — a Portland, Oregon, corporation that sponsors programs in wellness for individuals and businesses. Katie's modeling job for us is topped only by the role-modeling of wellness she does for her clients.

Akana Ma works as an international trade attorney whenever he can't ski.

Noriko Hosoyamada lived in Japan for the first part of her life. She has been an airline stewardess, an interpreter, a quality manager, and is currently a pre-med student. She has translated for major corporations worldwide and is mastering the language of yoga in her spare time.

Index